Fusion Press
a division of
Satin Publications Ltd.
20 Queen Anne Street
London W1M 0AY
Email: sheenadewan@compuserve.com

Cover Image: Nickolai Globe
Layout: Justine Hounam
Printed and bound by The Bath Press Ltd.

©2000 Belinda Grant Viagas
ISBN: 1-901250-74-1

Just Quit!

Giving up Smoking the Holistic Way

Belinda Grant Viagas

Acknowledgements

Yvonne Worth was my good fairy in London. Dilys Guildford initially 'zapped' me and reawakened our friendship. Drs. Smita and Pankaj Naram informed my interest in Ayurvedic medicine. Ken and Beryl Meadows and my friend in the circle showed me how to remember everything. Ellen Lally, my grandmother, continues to bring a special joy to every Friday, and I treasure our time together.

Dedication

To Nora, my mother, who continues to lead the way.

Disclaimer

The exercises and therapies detailed in this book are suitable for normal healthy adults. The author, publisher, their servants or agents cannot accept responsibility for loss or damage suffered by individuals as a result of following any advice in this book. It is strongly recommended that individuals suffering from, or with a history of, high blood pressure, heart disease or any other medical condition, undertake demanding physical exertion only after seeking professional advice from their health advisor.

Belinda Grant Viagas, N.D., D.O., Dip.C., trained as a naturopath, osteopath and counsellor before starting work as a Natural Healthcare practitioner. She operates a postal advice service, and lectures and leads seminars and workshops around the world.

Other books by the author

Detox Diet Book

The A-Z of Natural Healthcare

Natural Remedies for Common Complaints

Natural Healthcare for Women

A Pocket Guide to Therapies

Nature Cure

Contents

Contents

Conversions into Imperial and Metric Measurements

Although many cooks still use the British Imperial weights and measures, Metric is fast becoming the accepted method in the kitchen. Imperial does not convert easily into Metric, and most recipe books round the resulting figures either up or down, to the nearest unit of 25g (almost one ounce).

Solid Weights

Imperial . . . . . . Metric recommended

Imperial	Metric recommended
1oz	25g
2oz	50g
4oz	100g
8oz (1/2 lb)	225g
12oz	350g
14oz	400g
16oz (1lb)	450g
2lbs 3oz	1000g (1kg)

Liquid Measures

Imperial . . . . . . Metric recommended

Imperial	Metric recommended
1/4 pint	150ml
1/2 pint	300ml
1 pint	600ml
1 1/2 pints	900ml
1 3/4 pints	1000ml (1 litre)

Spoon measures

Standard spoon measures are used throughout, and all spoonfuls are level measures except where specified.

1 tablespoon = 15ml spoon
1 teaspoon = 5ml spoon

Cup measures

These vary with the ingredient, although a general rule for the size of cup is one that contains 8 liquid ounces, 1/2 pint, or 300ml of liquid.

INTRODUCTION

Congratulations. If you have just quit smoking, you have made one of the greatest positive health decisions you will ever make. Continue your good work, and ensure you reap the benefits of not smoking, by maintaining your weight.

Just Quit! will guide you through the changes that you need to make to your eating patterns in order to reduce your inclination to return to the habit, and to reinforce your resolve, through using a range of natural methods. It has been designed as a comprehensive support for the varied challenges of this important time. The book concentrates on what is new and incoming, and encourages you to look forward to a healthy and harmonious future. It does not analyse your old habits, but presents you with a wide range of exciting possibilities for change.

If you are considering stopping smoking, but have been put off by the thought of gaining weight, then this book will also help. If you have been using the possibility of weight gain as an excuse, you have just lost another reason to procrastinate.

There are a number of incentives to encourage you to follow the *Just Quit!* diet, but the only really important one is your intention to succeed. This is a three step plan that concentrates on the most crucial things that your body will be needing: cleansing, energising, then balancing and revitalising. The diet works through a careful choice of foods, and when and how you eat them. It enables you to control your own nourishment and provides a strong structure that will contain appetite surges, cravings and mood swings. The diet will wake up your taste buds and is full of delicious meal suggestions that can become part of your ongoing system of healthy eating. You will also find an outline of the supplements that will be most useful, and how best to take them.

Just Quit! will enable you to focus on positive nutrition for your body, rebalance your energy, redress any blood sugar imbalance and reassess your attitude to your own nurturing and care. It is designed to support your best efforts, and is a lifestyle plan and a way of eating that will smooth the transition into non-smoking and eliminate weight gain. It includes a variety of natural, safe and effective measures to strengthen your resolve and work towards your success. All these have the added benefit of soothing jangled nerves, and restoring harmony to your body at this key time.

The chapter on reawakening our senses encourages the discovery of non-food treats and sensual pleasures as rewards and celebrations. These need to be included into your schedule on a regular basis. Natural remedies like aromatherapy oil baths and massages marry well with techniques for achieving inner calm through relaxation, meditation and guided imagery. Together they start to build a sense of specialness that carves a new way to positively care for yourself.

There are some obvious areas where natural remedies will be most beneficial at this time, such as essential oils that will work to reawaken your sense of smell, and then to delight it. Coughs, mucus congestion and other common ailments will respond very well to a non-chemical approach to healing, and you will soon be witnessing your own powers of self-regeneration. Making sure you express any surfacing emotions and effecting changed patterns in your everyday life, mean you can move on from this experience with a different perspective and a genuine sense of renewal.

Whatever your old patterns and habits are, food will be intimately connected, and yet it is one of the most powerful and immediate medicines you can use to reinforce the change in your life. Your diet can provide an effective and immediate way to redress health imbalances and ensure optimum energy levels. It is also a chance to repair the damage of repeated insults by focusing on putting something good in your mouth! Specific meals and ways of eating will help you slough off the residue of toxins in your system and give a quick fix to your health. You will be able to restore vitamin and mineral levels to ensure you have the peak energy and vitality you need. All the foods have been carefully chosen to maximise the special benefits you will need most at this time, and to minimise the incidents of cravings and feelings of loss.

The chapters on food explain how individual foods will help you, and you can use that information to build a personalised eating plan to meet your own individual needs. Alternatively, you can just follow the diet. It has been specially designed to take you through the first month as effortlessly as possible, rebuilding your basic health and addressing specific imbalances to ensure optimum performance. You will also find recommendations for changing your timetable, waking up your taste buds, staying calm, and a host of other measures that have been proven as strong, effective aids that will power you forwards into a future that is safely contained within good health habits.

This is all about caring for ourselves, honouring our wide range of needs and paying attention to our subtler senses. Learn how you can harness any nervous energy and use it to fuel your way through the uncertainty of this time of change, and find ways to respond and express your feelings more easily and fully. Keep the spirit of fire alive in your life and work to maintain your own inner body heat and passions. Transform your pattern of nourishment by changing the way you relate to the world around you, and analyse and meet the need for something to put in your mouth. Let the natural world support you as you reawaken your senses and use simple and effective natural remedies as safe and gentle healers to harmonise your body and your experience.

An holistic approach to managing this change in your life provides a host of different ways, techniques and methods for ensuring that you can harmonise and restore balance to your system. The energy of this time need not be about feelings of deprivation, it can be an opportunity to shake loose a range of habit patterns and start out on a new way of living that embraces an abundance of good things. A change like this rarely happens in isolation; the ramifications can be felt in all aspects of your life from sleeping patterns through to appetite and energy levels.

Just Quit!

When you focus on the benefits of positive change and self care, you can be too busy to bemoan the loss of any worn-out ways of doing things. There is a wide range of methods that are all worthy of exploration and, at the very least, they will relieve some of the more uncomfortable symptoms of change. You can choose to explore as many as you have time for, or select a few specific techniques to target your own special needs. The principles hold true for all types of old addictions, and can be transferred to other times in your life, and to other potentially stressful situations.

There is a lot to do, and there is no shortage of things to keep you busy as you focus on the power and transformative energy of change; working to manifest it in a myriad of practical ways. When you change the hooks that habits hang on, you dislodge the whole pattern of addiction and find space for something new. This book is intended to offer you support and encouragement through this time, and to provide some new suggestions for ways to make transition easier, and enable you to be successful in reaching your goals. You can read it through and explore all the tips and techniques, or turn to page 83, start the diet right now, and let the foods begin to do the work.

"Whatever you can do, or dream you can, begin it. Boldness has genius, power and magic in it. Begin it now." Goethe

GETTING STARTED

Just quit. Planning too much can become a reason not to do something – another delaying tactic, so seize the moment and begin your new positive health habits right now. Take a deep, cleansing breath, and as you release it, imagine any tension and disharmony leaving your body. Take another deep breath, and see anything you no longer need leaving your system as you slowly breathe out. Now you have done your first breathing exercise, and can use it to fuel you forwards into being clear in your intentions, and manifesting your desires. You can start by introducing different things into your regular schedule right away, and try some of the methods, techniques and food ideas detailed in this book. You may find, however, that the best results come from diving right in and changing your routine and your diet, and just quitting the old bad habits.

You will notice some physical changes almost immediately. Sometimes the energy for change that you release in your body will feel like it could overwhelm you. Do not be dissuaded from your purpose. Energy rushes are a positive sign that your body is freeing itself up from old patterns of behaviour and gathering the momentum for change. See these as an encouraging symptom, and welcome and use the surge of available energy. Start to enjoy the reawakening of physical sensations and your body's natural responsiveness. Feel your body supporting your decision to change as it de-stresses and sloughs off unwanted toxins, relaxing into a more comfortable posture as it manifests your desire.

If at first you gain a pound or lose a pound in weight, do not panic. Look to the long game, and support your body through this time of change. Any irregularities should settle down after a month of intensive self care. Implement the good food advice, or follow the diet, and you will balance your system and be able to maintain a natural weight for yourself.

All of the natural ideas, ways, means and remedies in this book will support you in achieving your goal; all you have to do is start using them today. Making a beginning is the most important thing you can do – after that the energy of change will carry you forward. Consider following the diet, or incorporating some of the food ideas because this is one of the most immediate ways you can influence your own biochemistry and effect a smoother transition into good health habits.

TIPS FOR SUCCESS

• Focus on what is new, incoming and positive, not on what has just left your life. Consider counting your blessings – listing five things you can be grateful for at the end of every day. Remember to include the magnitude of your capacity for change, your clear ability to manifest that, and your physical and emotional responsiveness to your own strong will.

• Stay warm. Keeping active is a good way to do this, but make sure that you stay well wrapped up too, and watch out for cold feet and hands throughout the day and at night. Choose warming foods that will heat you up from inside.

• Cultivate your own inner encouragement. Make sure that the voice inside your head is willing you forwards, stimulating your resolve and backing up your ideas. Find constructive ways to silence or distract any less than encouraging voices, and develop positive strategies to calm and soothe yourself right from the start.

• Maintain your feeling of being connected to Spirit in whatever personal way suits you best – return to a still, meditative inner space, say a prayer, and get close to positive smoke from fire, flame, smudge or incense (see page 61).

• Reward yourself with non-food treats to celebrate your successes. Every day that you manage to meet your goals and achieve positive things for yourself is worthy of celebration. Choose ways that will hold personal meaning for you, and invest time and energy in determining how best to do this.

• If you were to choose just one piece of advice from this whole book, pick the breathing exercises (see page 9), or the Taste Bud Treats (see page 85).

EMERGENCY FIRST AID

If you experience any panic or feel that your resolve is slipping, consider the following:

• Stop what you are doing right away so that you can focus on what you are feeling or experiencing. Walk away from your desk, put down the washing up, or switch off the television.

• Focus on where you are right now in this present moment. Reinforce this with a simple reality check – name five things that you can see, e.g. window, phone, book, etc., or voice three truths about yourself, e.g. I am 28 years old, I am wearing blue trousers, etc.

• Use a physical anchor (see page 54) to relax yourself physically and remind yourself what it feels like when you are calm, relaxed and in control.

• Take at least one very deep and full breath. This will cleanse your system, relieve any immediate cravings, and relax your body – relieving muscular tension in your neck and shoulders. It will also reaffirm your connection with the universal source of loving energy and deepen your own relationship with it.

• Do something physical to use the energy, e.g. go for a walk, even if it is just around the room; climb a flight of stairs; do some isotonic exercises.

Remember that this is a challenge, and the way that you meet it will define your personal success. The only standard of excellence you need to meet is the one that you choose for yourself. Other people's attitudes and opinions are their own business. If you want to be successful, then this book will help you focus your intention, and find ways to support your own best efforts.

LETTING AIR IN

Oxygen is one of the greatest aids you can use when it comes to redressing imbalances in the body and eliminating toxic residues. It seems too obvious to say that breathing is essential, but many of us do not breathe as easily or as fully as we need to, especially when we are tense or under stress. Smoking will have caused an irregular breathing pattern that will have established itself in your diaphragm, the main muscle involved in breathing. Remedying this is both easy and pleasurable. Breathing exercises will instigate new patterns of health and well-being, and exercise will ensure that your body is able to use this oxygen fully.

Simply stopping whatever you are doing, taking a deep, easy breath into your lungs, and then making sure you breathe all the way out again will buy you a moment in your busy schedule, top up your energy levels, and suppress any cravings you may have. It is one of the most effective and natural remedies you can find.

THE BREATH OF LIFE

A dramatic change needs to be made in the way your diaphragm works. You will have been used to an unusual breathing pattern for some time, one that resisted the body's natural flowing rhythm, but concentrated on a stop/start and holding motion. Re-educating your diaphragm through a variety of breathing exercises will enhance your feelings of well-being because you will be rebalancing your body as well as improving oxygen levels. Your body needs plenty of air to help in the cleansing process, and even your clarity of thought and will-power will be improved in line with your higher oxygen uptake.

With every full and relaxed breath that you take, your diaphragm should fall and rise in a strong wave that will serve to massage all the organs in your body.

As part of the body's physical cleansing, you may well find that you are experiencing coughs or chestiness. This is your body's way of clearing out any congestion or debris from your lungs and throat, and is a positive sign. Regular breathing exercises will power this cleansing and ensure a return to normal localised health.

Breathing exercises need to be done every day. The best time to do them is first thing in the morning, just after you wake up, and before rising and starting the day. This will reinforce your good intentions and help introduce a balanced breathing pattern from the start. There is a range of different breathing exercises to choose from, and all work with much the same end effect, so you can try them all and settle on a few that you like, or use a different one every day. When you are into the routine of using them, spending 5-10 minutes working with your breath each morning will be enough to balance you. Initially, though, you may choose to spend about 20 minutes each day with your exercises.

BREATHING EXERCISES

EASY NATURAL BREATHS

This basic breathing exercise builds a strong foundation for every breath you take. It will show you just how rhythmic and easy your breathing pattern can be, and will help you restore full function to your diaphragm.

Start by sitting up with a straight back and feet flat on the floor, or you may like to do this lying down. Place your right hand palm down, on your middle, close to your belly button, and let it relax so that it is lying there quite comfortably. You may need to prop your arm up with a cushion or pillow to allow it to relax fully. Place your left hand palm down, on your upper chest, just below your throat, in the centre. Again let it relax. Now just keep breathing. Do not try to breathe in any particular pattern, just breathe.

Notice what is happening with your hands. Your right hand may be completely fixed because your belly is not moving at all, whereas your left hand may be rising and falling with each breath. This is the most common pattern for people who take shallow breaths. You may also find that neither hand is moving much.

Once you have noted what is happening, concentrate on your diaphragm. This strong sheet of muscle is suspended below your rib cage, and would ideally move up and down in a wave of rhythmic movement fuelled with each new breath that you take. As your lungs fill with air, it will naturally push down into your belly, and return back up again as you empty your lungs. Imagine for a moment what it will be like when your diaphragm is free to move in this way.

Now relax, and take increasingly deeper and deeper breaths until you imagine yourself breathing in each time right down into your belly, and out again from the very centre of your body. Let your abdominal muscles relax and notice how your right hand rises and falls slightly with each breath. When you are breathing in a deep, relaxed way like this your left hand and your upper chest will scarcely move at all.

Continue breathing in this way for several minutes and you will set up a template that your body will remember and be able to return to during the day. You will also be experiencing a profound sense of relaxation and calm. You can use this technique whenever you feel yourself to be stressed or in need of some peacefulness. With regular use, you will soon be breathing in this way most of the time.

OBSERVED BREATHING

Sit comfortably with your back straight and your feet flat on the floor. You can lie down to do this, but it is so deeply relaxing that sleep is too real a possibility. Close your eyes, and begin by taking some full, easy and relaxed breaths, letting your diaphragm free up and begin a wave of movement within your body. Keep your breathing free, and notice your shoulders and any other tight areas start to relax and release their tension. Once you have established a gentle, easy rhythm of breathing and are feeling comfortable, begin to notice the point on your upper lip where your breath flows past on its way into and out of your body. Just put your awareness there and see what it feels like. Keep your breathing rhythm soft and fluid, and let yourself be aware of the point on your lip where your breath touches it.

Although this may seem strangely simple, being at that point which is outside your body but aware of the passage of your breath connects you in a very real way with the whole function of breathing. It will help you keep to a regular breathing pattern, and also yield some insights into the nature of your breathing and your sense of connectedness. You can keep breathing this way until you feel it is time to stop, or you may like to move the point of your awareness after a while, placing it on the end, or at the very top. of your nose on the inside. In all cases, just be aware of what is happening, do not try and make the sensation or feelings change in any way; simply observe and experience it.

CIRCULAR BREATHING

This is a wonderfully rich and joyous technique that will expand your whole awareness. It is called circular breathing because it is continuous, and because it allows you to experience every aspect of your breath, although it actually has four stages.

Begin by sitting with your back straight and your feet flat on the floor, or again you may like to do this lying down. Cover your belly button with the palm of your left hand, and place your right hand palm down on top. Relax and make yourself comfortable. You may need to prop your arms up with cushions or a pillow.

Close your eyes, take a few easy, relaxed breaths and settle yourself. Now take a deep breath in, and imagine it entering your body through your belly button. Your hands there act both as a physical reminder of this place, and as a filter so that nothing unwanted can enter your system. Breathe in for a count of four, and then hold your breath for a count of four. Do not strain, simply let yourself hold the tension. Then breathe out for a count of four, and imagine the breath leaving your body through the same point as it came in. Then count to four while you remain empty. Again, do not strain, just relax into the emptiness and experience it. Repeat the cycle, breathing in, holding the breath, breathing out, and staying empty – each to a count of four.

Count silently inside your head, or let a sound like your heart beat or a ticking clock guide you. Be sure to find your own rhythm. Keep this continuous, deeply healing breathing going for as long as you feel comfortable. It is tremendously settling, and can be used for a few minutes wherever you are in the day to calm and settle you. It is a powerful remedy against stress or nerves of any type. As part of your daily practice it will both ease and re-energise you and is a wonderful aid to meditation, restfulness and heightened awareness.

HEALING BREATH

This is a lovely technique which allows you to maintain a regular breathing pattern while using the power of your mind to harness your healing energy. Begin by getting comfortable, and either lying down or sitting with your back straight and your feet flat on the floor. Close your eyes and practice your easy, relaxed breathing for a few minutes to establish a good rhythm and aid your relaxation.

Now breathe out as deeply and fully as you can, and when you breathe in, imagine yourself breathing fresh, cleansing air right down into your body, as deeply as you can go. Repeat this a few times until you are feeling clear and any tensions, or tightness, disappear. With your next in breath, picture it reaching inside you to a point that lies just at the very tip of your spine. Breathe in as deeply as you can, and breathe out from the same point. Now visualise your breath as being full of clear, white light and carry it to the same spot, at the very base of your spine, as you breathe in deeply. Breathe out from that place, and be aware that a light still shines. Continue breathing into this place until the light that shines there is bright and clear. You may notice that it is coloured.

With your next breath, breathe in to a point deep inside you that is just below your belly button. Breathe out from there, and be prepared to carry some more clear, white light in to that place on your next breath. Notice how a tiny spot of light remains even as you breathe right out, and continue your rhythmic pattern of breath until the light that shines there is bright and clear. You may notice that it is coloured also, or that you are experience sensations of warmth or tingling. This is just fine.

Continue this breathing technique into your solar plexus, then your heart, your throat, and your forehead. Finally, when you are full of glowing light, take a few deep, clear breaths right up into the crown of your head and 'see' the light dropping down through your system until it reaches the base of your body before you breathe out from there. Continue this final breathing until your whole body feels alive and rejuvenated.

YOGIC BREATHING

This is just one of a vast range of Eastern breathing techniques that are associated with yoga practices. It is very useful for retraining the breathing mechanism, and also works to balance the system, improving left and right brain coordination and all cerebral function, as well as enhancing physical energy levels and well-being. When practised regularly it will have a steadying influence, although the initial effects can feel quite dynamic. It is important to do this in a measured, relaxed way, and if you feel dizzy or light headed take that as an indicator to stop and return to the exercise again the next day. Over time you will be able to increase the length of your yogic breathing.

Start by sitting comfortably with a straight back, and your feet flat on the floor. Close your eyes, and take some full but relaxed and easy breaths. Take a moment to focus on your breathing and the way the air moves into and out of your body.

Now, using your right hand, cover your right nostril with your thumb, and exhale through the left. Inhale again through the left nostril for a count of four, then close the left nostril with your ring finger so that both nostrils are closed and hold your breath for a silent, inner count of 16.

Release your right nostril and exhale fully to a count of eight, then inhale, again through the right nostril for a count of four. Close both nostrils and hold your breath for a count of 16. Release your left nostril and exhale to a count of eight. Maintain a sense of calm about these long counts – there is no race, and the more measured you can be the more beneficial the experience.

Complete the full sequence about 10 times, and then sit still, breathing deeply and easily for a few minutes before moving.

EXERCISE

You know you need to do more. We all do. Now more than ever your body will respond brilliantly to every extra minute that you spend using your muscles and enjoying movement. This is the perfect time to help your heart and speed elimination through some form of exercise, and your body will rarely be more receptive to finding ways to help itself be rid of the effects of smoking.

The key to exercise is to enjoy it. This means that if you like going to the gym, then this needs to be your first choice. However, there is an enormous range of alternative ways to increase your energy levels and improve your health. Walking is a brilliant all-round exercise that will increase your stamina, please your heart, and help keep your metabolism moving at an optimum. You can walk just about anywhere at any time – up and down stairs at your office, to work and back, around the park, or up and down in your home if you cannot get out. Dancing, is a wonderful work-out for your whole body, especially if you really let yourself go. Consider something energetic like Salsa, Line dancing, Flamenco or Irish dancing. Even waltzes can be good exercise if you get out on the floor often. There may be a sport or group activity that you have always been interested in, and now is definitely the time to go for it.

Whatever you choose, make sure you take some exercise every day. Start with five minutes a day, and if this is walking to the corner shop and back, if it is five minutes more than you are used to, then your body will benefit. Over the next month, aim to increase the amount by just three minutes a week, until you are doing 15 minutes a day, every day.

If you have not really exercised before, you will soon discover the benefits in increased energy, improved metabolism, and the tremendous rush of feel-good chemicals that your body produces quite naturally in response to activity. You will feel the effects whether you decide to take up running, or choose a slower movement form such as T'ai Chi or yoga.

The following exercises can be used as stretches to help you prepare for exercise, or if you take your time with them, can be your five minutes a day for the first week. They work to increase the energy flow throughout your body, to open and strengthen it, as well as increasing flexibility. They are known in the East as the Eight Jewels, and are said to have originated in China in the 12th Century.

WARM UP

Loosen up your body and gently increase your oxygen intake with these two exercises that work your lower and your upper body. Keep your movements slow and gentle throughout, and move in a relaxed and meditative way. Always respect your body's ability to listen to any messages it is sending. Never expect to feel pain, burning or discomfort.

Begin by standing with your feet together and flat on the floor. Bend your knees slightly, and lean forward until your fingers can sit on the front of your thighs just above your knees. Fix your gaze on the floor about five foot in front of you. Keeping your knees together, move them clockwise to make a circle. Rotate about 12 times to the right, then 12 times to the left, taking at least three seconds for each circle. Build up over the next four weeks until you can make 30 circles in each direction. When you are finished, slowly straighten up and lower your hands to your side. If you are not used to exercise, you may hear some joint clicks as you move around. Stop if you feel pain, but otherwise, these should not be anything to worry you.

Warm up your upper body by standing with your feet about shoulder width apart, and bending your knees a little so that you begin to sit down, while keeping your back straight. Let your body dip by about 2-3 inches. Raise your arms and bend your elbows until your hands are in front of your chest, and prepare to make a breast-stroke type of swimming movement through the air. Stretch your arms out in front of you as you breathe out, and then sweep them around to your side and back in front of your chest as you breathe in. Keep your breathing full, and your movements slow and relaxed. Complete about 12 of these, building up over the next month until you can do about 30. When you are finished, slowly straighten your knees and lower your arms.

THE EIGHT JEWELS

These stretch, tone and strengthen the body's main energetic pathways in turn, so do them in sequence, or choose those which feel most beneficial. Take your time, remember that this should be relaxing and enjoyable, and never strain, force yourself, or work through any pain or discomfort.

THE FIRST JEWEL

Stand with your feet shoulder width apart, and bring your arms up over your head. Turn your fingers in to meet each other with your palms facing upwards. Stretch your arms right up above your head with your finger tips almost touching and your hands flat and palm up all the time. As you do this, breathe out. Then bring your hands back down until they are just above your head, bending your elbows, and breathing in. Repeat this stretch and return eight times.

THE SECOND JEWEL

In the same stance, imagine you are holding a bow – stretch out your left arm to your side and bend up the hand so that the palm is facing away from you. With your right hand, make a fist as though you are holding the bow string, and then keep your left hand and arm steady as you pull back across your body with your right. Breathe out each time you pull the bow, breathe in as you relax. Complete one 'bow-shot' on your left, then turn and reverse the exercise so that you are pulling the bow string with your left hand. Do this eight times.

THE THIRD JEWEL

Stand as before, and raise your right arm over your head, keeping it straight. Bend your hand back so that the palm faces upwards, and bend your left hand so that the palm is facing down to the floor. Keeping both hands bent, slowly move one hand up while moving the other one down, alternating between right and left being uppermost, so that there are eight stretches in all. Keep the fingers on the top hand pointing backwards and those of the bottom hand pointing forwards. Breathe out as you stretch your hands apart, and in as you relax and swop hand positions to begin the next stretch.

THE FOURTH JEWEL

Stand as before and raise your arms up in front of your body to about chest height. Imagine that you are delicately holding a large balloon filled with air that sits between your hands and your chest. Keeping a gentle hold on it, turn at the waist, reaching slightly round to your right while your breathe out. When you have turned as far as you comfortably can, turn your palms outward. Then slowly return to the front, turning your palms back inward, and breathing in. Then turn to your left, and alternate turns until you have made eight. Keep your feet flat on the floor the whole time and your arms in a rounded position, so you do not burst the balloon!

THE FIFTH JEWEL

Stand as before, but shift your weight on to your right foot. Arc your right arm up over your head, and let your left heel lift of the ground slightly as you slowly and very gently bend over to that side. Let your arm curl over your head as it bends at the elbow, and keep it feeling heavy and relaxed. Let your head and neck relax as they lean into the bend, and try and feel like a piece of bamboo bending gently in the wind. Breathe out. Come back up very slowly, breathing in as you do, and then change to the other side and repeat until you have done eight bends.

THE SIXTH JEWEL

Stand as before, bring your arms up over your head, and then let them sweep gently down in front of you as you bend your knees and breathe out. Touch the outside of each knee with your slowly falling hands. (Think of a skier.) Hold that position for a second, and then stand up slowly, bringing your arms back up to shoulder height as you breathe in. Hold for a second, then repeat the exercise eight times.

THE SEVENTH JEWEL

Stand as before, and fold your thumbs inside your fists. Slowly extend one arm forward with your closed fist, palm down, while you draw the other one back to your side, palm up. Breathe out as you do this. Relax for a moment, then turn the fists over as you reverse the arms – reaching back with one, extending the other, and breathe out. At the end of each extension, squeeze your thumbs gently for a second. Then relax and breathe in. Make eight slow punches altogether.

THE EIGHTH JEWEL

Stand as before with the back of your wrists resting in the small of your back, one on each side of your spine. Use your knees to gently bounce yourself up and down, keeping your feet flat on the floor. Continue to keep your movements slow and easy. (Think of riding a horse.) Breathe out through your nose in short puffs as you bounce eight times, then take one smooth, long inhalation through your nose as you continue to bounce eight times. Complete eight full breaths (eight short out-puffs, and one smooth in-breath), bouncing all the time.

WINDING DOWN

This is as important as any other aspect of the exercise, and is a great way to give your body a moment or two to cool down. It will relieve any tension and help you settle your energy before you go on with your day.

Stand as usual, and make your hands into loose fists. Swing both arms together to one side, so that both your fists come at least as high as your shoulders, then let them swing down across your body, and up to the other side. Keep your movements weighty and long, but as vigorous or languorous as feels right for you. Make at least 12 full swings.

Rest your hands on your hips. Move your feet together and keeping them flat on the floor, rotate your hips about six times first to the right, then around to the left. Keep your head still, and try not to lean forward or backwards, just let your pelvis do the work.

Just Quit!

Let your arms settle back to your side, and stand still for a moment, feeling the difference in your energy, and letting yourself settle before you move on.

REAWAKEN
YOUR SENSES

There is a wide and wonderful range of natural ways to bring your body back to a magnificent awareness and alert appreciation of life that involves all your senses. Dulled taste buds and a long lost sense of smell can be transformed into sources of great joy, and your sight, hearing and touch skills can all be very pleasurably enhanced using a range of pleasant and effective natural healthcare methods and remedies.

TASTE

Be prepared for things to taste very differently to you over the next few weeks. If there are foods you never had much of a liking for, now is the time to try them again. Favourites can become less than exciting, and you might also find yourself yearning for different or new and more exacting flavours. Your taste buds will be ready to be reawakened and this is one of the most pleasurable experiences. You will be able to rediscover the layers of taste and flavour contained in the most simple meals, and the intense pleasure this can generate. Taste buds that have been battered and under-performing can be teased back to life quite quickly, and the benefits are enormous.

Just putting something onto your tongue will initiate a change throughout your body. If you doubt this, suck a slice of lemon and feel your eyes narrow, your toes curl and your gut tighten. Or eat a fresh peach and notice how your body softens and your breathing relaxes in response to the sweet nectar. This is one of the reasons that food can have such a profound effect on how your body works. It is not just the nutrition and the energy that is important but rather the initial reaction as well, and this is where your taste buds do their work. Beyond this, the consistency, texture and temperature of what you put in your mouth are also important. The joy of discernment can translate into maximum satisfaction with minimum input.

Stay relaxed when you put something in your mouth, take the time to experience it and savour the taste, letting the flavour linger on your tongue, pleasing your taste buds and satisfying your appetite. When food is rich and flavoursome, and we can discern and delight in the depth of that stimulation, there is no reason at all to bolt meals, or to overeat. If the taste buds are satisfied, then the appetite is too.

We can all recognise sweet tastes, and savoury, but there is a range of other tastes that all benefit the body in their richness and variety. It is good to include all of these as part of your taste stimulus every day. This also offers you a new way to look at balancing your diet, ensuring that you get a good mix of the different tastes without over dependence on any one.

Sweet is an obvious taste that we can all recognise, but it is worth looking for the subtle sweetness that is present in cooked rice, squash and onions as well as the more up-front fruit and other sugars. Sweet taste is such a treat for the body, it deserves to be respected and added in very small amounts.

Salt is another instantly recognisable taste that adds a little spice to our life – it works to bring out the other flavours in any meal. Explore the layers of saltiness that come from table salt, then the fuller taste of sea salt, and the enticing promise of saltiness in seaweeds and sea vegetables. A little salt goes a long way, and it is a shame to abuse this wonderful taste by overindulging. Salt is added to so many meals and packaged foods that we can soon develop an over-reliance on it, and you may need to remove it from your diet altogether for a short while to remember just how lovely a little of it really is.

Sour tastes in moderation will stimulate digestion and add savour to meals. Think of the tiny amount of vinegar or lemon juice you need to add to a salad dressing to make it spark, or the slight edge that a yoghurt marinade will give to a dish. Sour tastes bring an element of reality into your experience, but too much can lead to a sense of 'turning sour' and becoming jaded.

Bitter is the taste of tonic water and is found in spring greens and chicory. A little of it clears the senses and cleanses the palate. This can also have a debilitating effect if taken to excess, being somewhat chilling, but a small amount adds a definite frisson to a meal.

Pungency is found in the heat of black pepper and spices, and also in mustard, garlic, radishes and ginger. Think of how garlic adds something to a meal, but a whole dish might be too much. Pungent tastes encourage the body to express itself and instigate cleansing. See this for yourself when you eat something hot and spicy and all your mucus membranes begin to decongest – your sinuses clear, your eyes may water, etc.

Astringent is the taste that makes your mouth dry and puckered, and it continues this effect throughout your digestion. Pomegranates have some astringency, as do crab apples and cranberries. It is also discernible in beans and potatoes. This tends to dampen the fire of chillies, and of over enthusiasm, and brings you back to yourself.

Turn to the Taste Bud Treats on page 85 to see how useful your sense of taste can be in deepening your resolve for change and effecting new habits in your life. Using these treats daily will wake up your whole system and galvanise your efforts.

SMELL

If you have been around a lot of smoke, the delicate mechanisms in your nose will be fairly battered, and your sense of smell will have receded as a protective measure. Reawakening it opens up your world to a multitude of pleasures that can appear instantly and transform your life. Smell is as important as taste in order to enjoy your food and begin the process of digestion. Smell and memory are intimately connected, and you can realise this for yourself when the scent of barley sugar takes you back to the early days of your childhood, or when a waft of scent reminds you of your lover. Smell is a powerful force. Teasing it back will augment and enhance your experience beyond measure as it regularly delights you. Place yourself in situations where you can re-experience this wonderful scent; expose yourself to sea air that is scented with its salty mist, and visit gardens for the multitude of delicate perfumes released by the flowers. A gentle breeze can carry wafts of scent from far away to tantalise your senses and your memory, and you can ensure that you are surrounded by a palette of uplifting aromas through your own efforts.

You may find that some of your current choices about smells change during this time. Favourite perfumes may no longer please, and new scents may become more appealing. This is likely to vary and will come and go for a while, but over time your sense of smell is likely to be improved. You now have the chance to improve your discernment and expose yourself to the greatest possible range of attractive scents and aromas. Make sure they are as positive as possible, and take every opportunity to indulge this sense. Follow your nose in a florist or garden centre, and open yourself up to a whole range of delights. Smell the foods you buy, and bring to your kitchen the rich, heady perfume of ripe peaches, the powdery promise of field mushrooms, and the heavy aromatherapy of freshly crushed sweet basil leaves. Bake some whole garlic cloves and inhale deeply their pungent medicine.

Extend this into the rest of your home by keeping fresh flowers, or flowering plants such as jasmine near you. Rosemary has a beautiful flower, and its strong woody scent is excellent for clearing the mind and enhancing memory. Roses, too, have a unique soft, powdery perfume. Substitute these, pot pourri and essential oils for chemical air fresheners and strong detergents.

Aromatherapy is becoming increasingly well known. Though most commonly linked with massage, this is a wonderful way to treat your whole self, as well as pleasing and encouraging your nose. You can use essential oils to fragrance your rooms as well as to treat your body, and to fill your life with the blessed fragrances of herbs, woods and flowers.

Aromatherapy oils are concentrated essences that are extremely potent, and you will never need more than 2-3 drops to achieve your desired effect.

Deter insects by adding a few drops of citronella to a candle for burning in a window, or out of doors. Sweeten a room by wiping the surfaces with a damp cloth on which you have sprinkled a few drops of bergamot essential oil. Use dilute lemongrass essential oil to disinfect and to ground you with its unique citrus smell. Spray diluted ylang ylang onto your bed sheets to add a spicy, sensual aroma to your nights, and add a few drops of thyme to an incense burner or diffusion ring to ward off coughs and colds.

Add two drops of lavender to a warm bath to balance and re-energise you, or add two drops of black pepper oil to a foot bath to warm and stimulate you after a long day. Mix essential oils together in a base or carrier oil such as olive or sunflower, and develop your own perfumes. Never put the essential oils directly on to your skin because they can burn.

NASAL MASSAGE

Give yourself regular nose treats by indulging in the luxury of wonderful smells. Reinforce your nasal health at this special time by massaging morning and evening with a little oil. Make sure your little finger is quite clean and that the nail is short. Pick up a dab of olive oil or ghee with it and very slowly and carefully insert it into your nostril. Do not push. Let it work its way up as far as is comfortable using small, slow, circular movements. Rotate your finger first in a sunwise circle, and then reverse it as you slowly let your finger slip out. Repeat with your other nostril. When you do this slowly and carefully it is extremely soothing and will settle your whole system as well as improving your sense of smell.

If you find your sense of smell is not responding to these delicious stimuli, you may like to consider a couple of natural remedies that may redress the situation.

Take a Zinc supplement. The easiest and best way to do this is to suck Vitamin C lozenges that contain Zinc. Follow the directions on the tub, it is important to make sure you always have them after food. Take the maximum dose for 3-5 days. If you notice an improvement during this time, then continue taking or seek out a specific Zinc product to supplement your needs. Take this for one month, having one day off each week. This enables your system to rest and to find balance, so reducing dependency.

Tissue Salts are available in chemists and health food stores, and work to rebalance the body biochemically. Nat. Mur. is an especially good remedy for restoring the sense of smell. Tissue Salts are taken as small lactose tablets. Take them as directed on the tub, and be sure not to touch the tablets, but to decant them into the lid and put them directly onto your tongue. Leave a gap of at least 20 minutes between taking anything to eat or drink and having a dose of Tissue Salts to make sure they are fully absorbed. Take half the recommended dose for five days. (Your body will be extra sensitive at this time, so it is best to start conservatively.) If it has been beneficial and you want to continue, take the full dose for a further five days. Rest for two days, and repeat this five days on, two days off pattern for the rest of the month.

SIGHT

Your eyes are the most obviously magnificent and beautiful reflection of your mind. They pick up everything that goes on around you and relay it directly on for you to discern, process and decide upon. They also express your thoughts and feelings, often more immediately and eloquently than you can with words.

For some time now your eyes will have been suffering repeated smoky insults, and they, and the skin around them, will respond brilliantly to some loving care.

WAKING UP YOUR EYES

When you wake each morning, gently exercise your eyes. You can do this before you get out of bed and it will be just as effective. With your eyelids shut, look up inside your head. Then move your eyes as far as they will go to the right, then down towards the rest of your body, and over as far as they can to your left, then back up again. Hold the extreme of each movement for the count of five. Then reverse the circle, moving first to your left, then down, etc. When you have made a complete circle in each direction, open your eyes and slowly do it again, holding each position for a count of five.

Your eyes have a lot of work to do each day, and simply closing them for a moment or two will often be enough to refresh them. Shifting your focus from time to time will ensure that the muscles that surround the area do not become too tense. Do this easily by looking away from what you are doing and resting your gaze on something across the room, then looking out of the window, and then down to your hands. This takes you from the middle to the far distance, and then back into close up. You only need to hold each range for a moment in order to benefit.

DEVELOPING INNER VISION

For a fully relaxing treat, sit at a table or desk and rest your elbows upon it. Let your head sit heavily in your hands as your palms cup over your eye area. Relax, and feel the warmth from your hands spreading over and into your eyes. Make sure your hands shut out all the light. Now take a few deep, easy breaths, and relax as fully as possible. Re-run a beautiful scene, event or journey in your mind's eye, making it as vivid, colourful and life-like as your memory will let you. Observe all the detail and the sense of the place or occasion, remember how the light was, and how bright the colours were. Take your time, and make your experience as full and enjoyable as possible. The longer you spend reviewing your inner vision, the more rested your eyes will be when you open them again, so do not rush. When you are quite ready, remove your hands and hold your head up, open your eyes and blink five times. Then hold your eyes open for the count of five, and shut your eyes again for a minute. When you open your eyes again you should find them clear and focused.

Make sure that what you see is as beautiful and stimulating, and as bright and vibrant as it can be. Consider repainting the walls, or adding some splashes of colour to your home, workplace, and yourself, with accents and accessories. A brilliantly coloured cushion cover can provide a strong focus for a corner of the home or office, and a new scarf or pair of gloves is an inexpensive way to colourise yourself. Get out into the natural world – let your eyes revel in the beauty of a sunrise occasionally, and keep regular dates with areas of outstanding natural beauty.

Give your eyes a rest from too much screen use – have a break from television or take some time off if you work with a VDU. And take city eyes off regularly for a day in the countryside, or to a local park, where the soothing natural shapes and colours will rejuvenate you.

Use an infusion of the herb eyebright to restore sparkle and energy to tired eyes. You can buy this already made up into a cream, or make a wash yourself by adding one teaspoon of the dried herb to a mug of boiled water. Steep for 10 minutes, then soak two cotton wool balls in the liquid and use them to gently bathe your eyes. Squeeze the liquid down over your closed eyes, and when the cotton wool is no longer saturated, rest each pad over your eyes while you relax. You can keep this in the fridge for a cooling and refreshing eye mask to put on at the end of the day.

SOOTHING MASSAGE

Keep the skin around your eyes supple and relaxed by massaging very gently with a little light oil such as olive, sunflower or sesame. Dip your ring fingers into it and place them in the inner corner of your eye socket just beneath your eyebrow. You will find a small depression there, and can begin by using the lightest of pressure upwards and inwards on this point. Then trace a large, loose circle around your eyes moving delicately out along your brow and then underneath your bottom eyelid. Return to the starting point using a light, gliding, continuous movement. Do not use any pressure at all or you can damage the delicate skin around your eye. Let the oil and the warmth from your finger make this a gliding motion that lubricates and re-energises the whole area. Make five or six slow circles, and repeat this exercise morning and evening.

SOUND

You can use sound to calm and relax yourself – it is perhaps the most powerful stimulus that we respond to almost without realising. Consider for yourself the way you respond physically to the sound of running water, or the soothing tones of a familiar voice. Music has a very real potency. Regardless of its volume, the beat of music can influence your mood and agitate, excite, soothe and settle you. Since the start of time people have responded in the most profound way to the simple beat of a drum. It is used by Shamans to enter other realms of awareness, and by mothers who soothe their babies by holding them close to their heart.

Consider the sounds of nature – when did you last really listen to something that you enjoyed and that soothed and calmed your spirit. There are few things more restful than the rhythmic sound of the ocean's waves gently lapping onto a shore; or more calming than the gentle, scattered pattern of raindrops falling to the ground; or the voice of the trees as they dance with the wind. If you cannot travel to those places and hear those soothing sounds physically, then you can use your powerful imagination alongside one of the many recordings that you can buy, and have a relaxing and truly rejuvenating experience.

Hearing, paying attention and listening to things are all skills that we can develop. Not listening is just another way of switching ourselves off and keeping ourselves safe and free from harm. Unfortunately it does not actually work, because not listening properly simply robs us of another level of awareness that will actually augment and enhance our experience. Ask yourself how good your listening skills are – and on what level? Do you have good social skills that allow you to converse easily with others through listening as well as talking? Ask yourself occasionally if you have really heard what someone is trying to tell you. Sometimes the most generous gift we can make another is to really listen to them and witness what they are saying. And do you have the ability to listen to your own inner thoughts and feelings? Practice really hearing what is going on around you, and wake yourself up to the world out there with the following exercise.

EXPANSIVE LISTENING

Sit comfortably in a place where you will not be disturbed. Quiet your breathing and calm yourself until you are feeling settled and still. Close your eyes. What do you hear? Really listen to the layers of sound that surround you. Expect to be aware of the noise of the nearby traffic, but listen too for the gentle hum of electricity or phone lines, the sweet song of birds nearby, and the gentle buzz of insects flying by. Listen for passing sounds like a plane flying overhead, or a snatch of conversation from passers by. Pay attention to the sounds that your body is making – the soft swishing sound of your breath, the perfect beat of your heart, and any gentle gurgles and rumbles from your gut. Even when we choose a quiet place, the levels of aural stimulation are awesome, and this is a wonderful way to experience some of the things we normally filter out of our awareness.

Now take a deep breath, and hold it for a second while you reach for silence. Breathe out, and relax, bringing your senses back to their normal level of awareness, and taking a moment to re-orient yourself. Breathe easily for a moment or two before opening your eyes and moving on.

Make time every day to listen to your own inner voice that speaks of your true needs and desires. Enhance the satisfaction value of your sense of hearing. Turn up the volume if you need to, and increase the number of good sounds you listen to. Avoid noise, it is distracting and unsettling. Whether your choice in music is Vivaldi, M People or birdsong, do not leave it as background sound all the time, let it fill your head on occasion and really move you.

TONING

This is an exercise that will help you express yourself and expel any disharmony. It is remarkably simple to do, and is extremely successful in changing your energy, and that of the place you are in. It is enormously pleasurable, and you can do it every day for the pleasure it brings, incorporate it into your meditation practice, or use it as a form of self expression. It is a profoundly effective way of manifesting change in your body and in your humour, and you will often feel lighter, clearer, more peaceful or happier after doing it. Working with the breath in this way fills your body with oxygen, and allows you to experience making your own unique sounds. On a physical level it works to clear the sinuses and the chest, deepens and relaxes the breathing, and delivers a blast of usable energy from all that oxygen. Choose a place where you will not be disturbed, and cannot be overheard by others. Sit comfortably and take a few deep relaxing breaths. Choose a vowel sound (ah, ay, ee, o, oo, etc.,) and take another deep breath in. As you breathe out, let the air come out with the sound you have chosen. Do not worry about the pitch or the tone, or try to achieve any continuous sound or projection; just let out the sound. Then breathe in again straight away, and as you breathe out, let the air come out with the sound again. It might be noticeably different, and that is fine, or it may sound quite similar. Keep your breathing continuous. You will find that the note you are singing and the sound you make will change as you continue this exercise. You can let your body lead you in modulating the sound the way it needs to. It will eventually sweeten or harmonise, and by the time you are ready to finish you will be making and hearing the healing tones that your body needs to rebalance itself.

TOUCH

Every inch of skin that covers your body is alive with a multitude of receptors to record every nearby movement, each actual touch, and the slightest change in temperature. As an organ, your skin is remarkable in its size, ability, elasticity and sensitivity. We witness its healing powers every time a small cut or graze heals, or a spot disappears, and it is a valuable channel of elimination for the body.

As a receiver, the skin is more sensitive than a radio antenna. When you place your hand on someone's arm in greeting, your brain will be recording a host of information about how relaxed they are, and this skill can be used to benefit and help settle your own system. Using your own comforting touch is a wonderful way to restore the integrity of your link with your body.

Massage is an excellent way to communicate with yourself, or with another, and is a great way to feel in touch with your body. It will also meet the need for contact and the thirst for touch which we all have. Massage is an exquisite sensual pleasure as well, and can bring delight and joy to your whole body. You can do it simply and effortlessly as part of your bathroom routine. When you shower or bathe, use a moisturised soap or body wash, and make sure you cover your whole body with gentle or stimulating massage strokes.

MORNING MASSAGE

You can use massage to wake yourself up in the morning, and to soothe your way into sleep last thing at night. First thing in the morning, massage your head by rubbing it all over using your fingertips and the flat of your hands. Imagine you are giving your head a good shampoo, and vary the degree of pressure and the direction of your rubbing. Be as vigorous or as gentle as you feel is appropriate, and see how just a few moment's attention will wake you up and prepare you for getting up. Once you are sitting up, massage your feet too. You do not need anything except your hands in order to hold and massage your feet. This will wake up your whole system and leave you feeling very connected, as well as ready for the day.

Begin by sandwiching your foot between your hands for a moment to warm it. Then slowly knead the soft, cushioned skin of the ball of your foot, and increase the movements to sweep along the arch and down towards your heel. Run your fingers in between your toes, and then down over your instep and around your ankle. Make the sweeping movements long and relaxed. Finish by just stroking down the top of your foot towards the toes, and then along the sole of your foot towards the heel. When you are finished, and your foot feels tingly, alive and warm, hold it again between your hands for a moment or two before going on to wake up your other foot. Enjoy the experience. Approach your body with the attitude of a new lover – exploring every nook and softness with a tenderness and real care, and delighting in each new discovery. Let this be a source of real nourishment for yourself ever day.

EVENING MASSAGE

In the evening, use a drop or two of massage oil, or a few drops of olive or any other oil from your kitchen, to gently stroke away the cares of the day and prepare you for sleep. Dip your first two fingers into the oil and stroke across your forehead from the midline out to the temples. You can do this when you are lying down, and you may find this even more relaxing. Make a few strokes with each hand, and then add a little more oil to your fingers and make small, light circles around your temples. Let the movement be rhythmic and slow, and enjoy how your fingers glide loosely over your skin cooling and relaxing, and removing any worries and cares. Gradually increase the size of the circles so that you include a larger area reaching up into your hairline, and down over the top of your ears. When you feel relaxed, cup your hands over your ears, letting the warmth from them comfort and soothe you, and finish your massage like this.

Having a treatment from a professional massage therapist is a good way to relax and enjoy your body. You will also be able to pick up some tips from the way they work that you can use for yourself. Ideally, though, you will be too involved in the experience to let your mind trace too many techniques or methods. Having massage is a real treat. It allows you to benefit from a warm and caring touch that can offer a full spectrum of health enhancing benefits from increasing your relaxation to nurturing you emotionally. In our society, touch is rarely shared except between lovers, and within the family between parents and children. Being naked, or nearly naked, with another person who is looking after you is a really trusting thing to do, and can help to repair any early bonding issues or other emotions that have not yet resolved. On a physical level massage will also help your body to slough off toxins and rebalance itself.

Make some time each day for nakedness – let your skin breathe and enjoy the feel of a soft sheet against your body, or the rough fibres of a carpet, and appreciate the silky strength of wood as you lean against it. This has a myriad of therapeutic benefits; encouraging your skin function relieves pressure on other routes of elimination and is an enormously pleasurable treatment. It is good to feel the air brushing against your whole body as you move, and to become aware of the multitude of sensations that we can be open to just by simply being. If the weather is warm, stand near an open window and feel the fresh breeze touch you all over. In the colder months, turn up the heating for the evening and relax in the warmth and nurturing of your own nest.

GETTING TO THE POINT

There are special points on your body where your energy is more accessible, and Acupressure and Shiatsu are among those Eastern techniques that work with these energy points to stimulate or calm the system. Do this for yourself using a gentle pressure with your thumb: Feel for the point in between your thumb and first finger right up towards your wrist where the bones meet. This point is called 'Meeting Mountains', and the valley that exists between the two bones is an excellent point to use to relieve a headache. Hold your hand with your other hand, and let your fingers support its weight. Simply press down on it with your thumb, holding each pressure for about a second, and then release and repeat. Make your contact firm enough to be felt, but never use enough pressure to hurt or bruise yourself.

Other good points to use for yourself include one in between your nose and upper lip, right in the middle. Press this with your thumb and hold for five seconds, then repeat twice more for an instant energy lift. Find another point on your feet, in between your big toe and second toe. This mirrors the point on your hand: Find it by feeling in between the two bones in the fleshy part of your foot. Use your thumb and index finger as gentle pincers to stimulate this point. Press with your thumb once a second for five seconds to improve circulation, and to help warm up your hands and feet. All of these techniques invite you to get to know your body better, and can be enjoyed for the satisfaction of doing this, as well as for their specific helpfulness and efficacy.

FEEDING YOUR NEED

Your mind and body are intimately connected; the link between how you feel physically, and how you feel emotionally, is powerful and strong. Becoming conscious of your habit patterns, and what your feelings and emotions are, will help you release this addiction and strengthen your resolve. It will also deepen your understanding of yourself, and thereby enhance your effectiveness in the world.

Becoming conscious of what you are doing will help you through any energy rushes or surges of needy feelings. If necessary, stop whatever else you are doing so that you can concentrate on yourself for a moment, then remind yourself of where you are right now. You might need to say something reassuring to yourself to keep you in the moment, such as "I am 29 years old and sitting at my own office desk" or "It is Friday afternoon and I am on my way home". Stay calm. Take a deep, cleansing breath, and you should find that the urge has passed.

You might think that you are wanting something to eat all the time, but that is not actually so. You will have a strong habit of putting something in your mouth very often, perhaps several times every hour. If you start eating at that rate you will put on weight, and only succeed in switching the addiction from one substance to another.

Watch yourself for a while, inhabit the place inside you that is purely an observer on your life, and record your feelings as well as your actions, without getting caught up in them. Just for a few minutes, become conscious of what happens to you when you notice the desire to reach for a piece of food, or a sweet, or whatever. When does that desire come – is it in response to some emotional stimulus? Often our habits will include masking our feelings and will be a useful tactic to buy time or create a very real smoke screen that we can take some shelter behind. See if you can spot the emotions that generate your need for comfort – to put something in your mouth. Often these are the ones we find most difficult or uncomfortable, such as anger, grief, or maybe general feelings of low self-esteem or lack of confidence. Getting to know your feelings is a powerful step towards being in control of your life.

Rather than continuing to suppress these feelings, now is the time to realise them and to start creating a new you – a person with renewed self confidence, who is not afraid of their emotions, and knows how to use and express them appropriately. Practice on your own to start with, and then extend your range to include the other people in your world. You may feel shy initially, but confidence will soon grow. It might help to know that most people feel awkward about their feelings at some time in their lives, and many do not have as much confidence as it might appear.

Often, simply saying what you feel, e.g. 'this feels awkward' or 'I just don't know what to do' will be a tremendous relief to others who might also be feeling the same way, but do not know how to find the courage to say so. There may be people in your life who would benefit or learn something from any righteous anger that you have towards them, or it might fuel your way out of a truly difficult situation – remember that anger can be constructive too.

Dungeon theory is a good explanation for the way we often relate to feelings. If we encounter something that scares us, that is daunting in some way, or that we do not want to take the time to deal with, or do not have the resources for, we tend to lock it away in our own personal dungeon. Every time we think about what is down there, we reinforce our feelings of dread, fear or inability to cope. As a result, when we go near the place we re-double the lock on the dungeon door, reinforce the guard, or build greater, bigger and better defences. Soon that place can be air tight sealed and guarded better than any other structure on earth. This consumes a tremendous amount of energy, and a lot of time goes into checking that all the protection is in place, even after many of the actual responses have become automatic.

Finding the courage to walk past somewhere that is so well defended can sometimes seem daunting, let alone deciding to walk right in. What is important to remember, is that we are not the same person who first constructed the dungeon, and what we put in there also has its own life cycle. Sometimes when we revisit an experience, there is not actually anything there except the dust of memory. Remember how big everything and everyone appeared to be when you were a child? If you had encountered a Father Christmas before you were old enough to realise that he was wholly a good thing, you might have been frightened by his size, his bright red suit, and all that beard. If you had access to a dungeon, he would have certainly been one of its first inhabitants. Imagine how pleased he would be if you were able to go back and free him now.

There may be many things which might have seemed threatening to you when you were emotionally younger that you may now be able to release and see differently.

BURIED TREASURE

Think back to the time in your life when you first began smoking, and see if you can identify any particular feelings that were around or surrounding you at that time. Perhaps you were aware of anger that you could not find another way to express, or that you were anxious about changes that were occurring in your life and felt powerless in their wake. Maybe you had a sense of loneliness and felt excluded, and experienced a strong desire to join in with others. This is the perfect time to review those feelings and to find new ways to deal with them. Making emotional pain physical is a very common way of coping with something that we cannot understand, or can find no other way to deal with. Some things are just too painful to feel, so we seek other ways to divert ourselves from feeling that pain, often generating another type of pain that we can hope to have some element of control over.

Up until now, every aspect of your day has supported your habit, or has at least intimately been involved in it. Stopping the habit is central, but it also makes sense to actively change the situations, structures and ways that have contained and supported that habit. For the time in your life when you have done it, that was the best you could do. Now you have the opportunity to do it differently, and it is important to consider a few basic facts:

- Any pain that you might feel by remembering cannot be any worse than the pain you feel by knowing and not remembering.
- You have the power – you are proving it – to change your life, and this applies to every area of your world. You have chosen to stop employing certain negative habits that reinforce a self-sabotaging plan, and are now free to make moves, plans and to develop strategies that will forward your progress in every way and enable you to live the type of life you want for yourself.
- Follow your own inner timing, and develop trust and confidence in yourself.

It is time to recognise that a deep inner change has occurred and to recognise a new goal – that of furthering your own well-being. Now you have the opportunity to stop avoiding any painful feelings and begin to actively make choices to further a healthful and happy life for yourself.

Even if you are usually comfortable and secure in your feelings, this dramatic change to your lifestyle can give you the opportunity to review and deepen your exploration of your own emotional resource. Sometimes old feelings and memories will surface, and this is a chance to clear out any excess baggage. Consider emotion as Energy (E) in motion, and let it flow.

LIFE STRATEGIES – A PRACTICAL EXERCISE

Are you happy? Does your life work for you? Choose some major areas of your life and analyse them, e.g. Home, Work, Relationships, Social life and Health. There will be many overlaps, but take a good look at every aspect of each category, making it as broad as possible. Relationships, for example, will embrace your feelings about the loved ones in your life, your relationship with yourself, with people who have influenced you in your life up to now, and with the Creator.

Identify for each category:

• How happy you are in this area of your life?
• How you would like it to be?
• What changes would benefit you and support the way you want your life to be?

Then you can start to plan what changes you might like to make and begin to implement them. Even small changes can make a profound difference to the quality of your life. You can start making more time for yourself by taking just 10 minutes every day to be alone and keep a journal, or catch up with your feelings. (see page 40). You can positively influence your health by getting up 30 minutes earlier so that you are able to relax and have breakfast every morning. And you can make beneficial changes to your home by resolving to wash up at the end of every day, or by sorting out one cluttered cupboard, and improve your work life by instigating an empty desk policy.

Larger changes can be worked towards and achieved by making small goals and using each one as a stepping stone to the main prize. Remember that every day you can be actively involved in implementing your own plans for your future.

IDENTIFYING FEELINGS

Make a list of feelings and emotions. Make it as comprehensive as you can, and include as many different types as possible, whether or not you have any direct or personal experience of them. Be sure to include anger, resentment, joy, peace, grief, love, contentment, excitement, forgiveness and surrender. Now jot down one way of expressing the feeling next to each entry on your list. This does not need to be too considered or profound, just write down whatever occurs to you, and do not worry about repetition. You might put down 'throwing things' by anger; 'crying' by grief; 'dancing' by joy, etc.

When you are finished, review your list and consider how many of these feelings and emotions are really familiar to you, and which ones you feel most at ease with. From the vast range that is available to us, we often feel comfortable expressing just a few. See if you can broaden your emotional palette by exploring further. You may also like to experiment with some of the different means of expression and see how appropriate and easy each one feels. Return to your list from time to time to update and alter it, and keep it as a guide.

KEEPING A JOURNAL

This is a great way to explore your feelings and emotions and will help you identify your own inner agenda. It can also prove to be a good anchor during times of change and uncertainty. Looking back over your journal entries will help you record the cycles and themes that run through your life, and may well surprise you as you discover just how capable and multi-faceted a being you really are. Choose a special, bound volume to write in, or open a file on your computer – whatever feels most natural. Make an appointment with yourself each day to spend some time acknowledging and recording your feelings, and make sure that you keep it.

In the beginning you may need to encourage yourself to start writing, perhaps by trying to fill a page each day. Keep to this discipline, even if you end up writing about how hard it seems to write about yourself; how daunting the page looks with all its expectation and pressure. Do not worry – you can just write down the stream of thoughts that are in your mind, even if they seem disjointed and do not make immediate sense. Very quickly, this resistance will ease and you will find yourself developing a strong and rewarding communication that will allow your deeper feelings to be aired. Keep your journal private until, and unless, you decide you would like to share it with someone else. This will allow you total freedom to express and explore whatever you want.

If your sleep pattern is disturbed and you find yourself waking in the night, write down whatever is churning through your mind. Often, in the small hours of the morning, perspective gets the short shrift. However, by writing down your thoughts at this time you may discover some real insights, as well as relieving any anxiety, and so enable sound sleep to return.

Do not limit your self expression to words – if you want to use graphics to illustrate a point, or feel inclined to use drawings, paintings or sketches. Make space for them and allow this aspect of yourself to develop. You may also like to begin keeping a record of your dreams, or day-time fantasies. Feel free to explore any and all parts of yourself and your experience in this personal and safe medium. Record your goals and achievements, your private thoughts and dreams, your individual successes and your innermost secrets, and you become actively involved in the richness of your life, and in determining your own future.

PLAYING WITH YOUR FEELINGS

Acting out your feelings and emotions is a good way to get to know them, and to experience what it feels like when you allow these feelings to surface. You can do this on your own first as this will enable you try them on for size, and to discover which feel most comfortable and easy for you. Everybody feels more at ease with some emotions more than others. This can change from season to season, as well as in response to growth and change in our lives. Some situations are also much easier to deal with, and to be honest in, than others. Every time you identify with a character in a film, become involved with a storyline in a book you are reading, or feel moved by the lyrics of a song, you have the opportunity to take that feeling just a little bit further, and to make it your own; experiencing the feeling and exploring it in a totally safe, solitary way. The exciting thing about this is that even though you are playing, or pretending, the emotion is real, and you gain worthwhile experience expressing sometimes difficult emotions. This can build into a valuable resource that will allow you to express your feelings more freely with others, and help you become more responsive and 'in the moment' in your everyday life.

Imagine standing in front of an audience and performing a song that moves you – perhaps then you would feel free to put some real emotion into it and use your body and your voice to express what was going on inside you. The elation you automatically feel when you sing out loud is incredible – a free fun-ticket that takes very little effort. Picture yourself in a scene from one of your favourite films – say the lines that the character speaks, or move the script along a little by developing the aspect you most want to experience. Books are also great sources of inspiration because they rely so much on our own imagination to colour and clothe the characters. As well as expressing yourself in this way, take note of the range of feelings and emotions you are exploring, and endeavour to make them as wide and full as possible. Remember not to sing the melancholy ballads without looking at what is making you sad. Then, try balancing it with something joyous.

Emotions are incredibly exciting, and feeling and expressing anger, joy, or even fear can be tremendously exhilarating and liberating. The adrenaline rush that often accompanies the release of these feelings means a surge of energy flows through the system, waking up your whole body and making you feel really alive. Once they begin to express their feelings, many people find release from problems such as lethargy and mild depression, anxiety, and even physical concerns like poor circulation. The body and mind work together, and freeing up energy anywhere in the system changes your entire experience of this synthesis.

PERSONAL APPOINTMENTS

Make a private appointment with yourself every day, and make sure that you keep it. This can be just five minutes when you wake up, or before the end of your day, when you have time to be still and to check in with yourself and your inner needs and desires. Do whatever feels most appropriate in this time – use it to take stock, perform a daily inventory, or re-run the events of your day. Often, especially when we are busy, we can leave loose strands of ourselves that tie up our attention, or find that there are feelings that have not been expressed or dealt with. Use this time to do whatever you need to do, whether it is thinking things through, or doing some wild crazy dancing. Do not limit yourself. This is the time when you can develop the most important relationship that you have in your life – your relationship with yourself. Just like every other relationship, it will deepen and become richer with time. If you feel comfortable in and with yourself, it is easy to relax and be natural as fully as you choose to be with others, and in every aspect of your life.

Get to know your feelings, and you uncover another magnificent aspect of yourself. So, next time you feel the need to put something in your mouth, consider why. When you can answer that, you can move on and use some of the suggested diversionary tactics to placate your body, while you work on the real causes. Stop and close your eyes, and then imagine the thing you were reaching for as though it was already in your stomach. Visualise how it feels – did you really want that? If the answer is yes, then go ahead and eat it – if not, find something else to do right away to take your mind off it, and enable you to get some satisfaction from another source.

NOT JUST FOODS

As we have already explored, there are a number of things you can do to divert your attention away from putting something in your mouth, and the range of possibilities open to you is really limited only by your inventiveness. You can gain a sense of satisfaction from achievement (try entering competitions, doing crosswords, meeting goals) communicating (singing, letter writing, chatting on the Internet or on the phone), creating (plant a seed, sew a sampler, plan a website), being brave (model nude for an art class, take up a new hobby, address a public meeting), and being intimate (letting someone close physically, sexually or emotionally). This is a wonderful opportunity for you to experiment with some new ways of being successful and achieving satisfaction in your life. If ever there was a list of things you want to do, now is the time to consider them. You might also like to try:

gardening or planting a window box, a patio tub, or getting an allotment
sprouting your own seeds and shoots
yoga, T'ai Chi or some other gentle exercise form
making things such as needlepoint and sewing, tapestry or bargello work

archery
learning to juggle
turning out your wardrobe
playing chess
dancing
learning a new language
decorating and making things
sign language
finger painting
puppetry
fencing
candle making
playing a musical instrument
painting with water-colours, or oils, or pastels
appliqué work
design – you could re-design the garden, your filing system, or how you use your kitchen cupboards.

REWARDS

Different things will be treats for different people, but whatever you choose, you must reward yourself for doing well and being success-ful for another day. That means succeeding in your resolve, following this diet, and achieving what you set out to do each day. If your life is generally bound by routine, then bunking off for a day is one poten-tially enormous treat. If you are caring for a young family, try and organise a few hours on your own to go to the cinema to see your choice of film. If you rarely get the opportunity to indulge your inter-ests, then attending a lecture, or going along to a talk or a class might be a treat for yourself. Or it might be something as simple as buying yourself a bunch of flowers. Shifting the focus onto non-food treats will be the best way.

Make yourself a ridiculously long list of all the treats you can possibly think of. Let your mind run freely through all your desires, and include everything, no matter how small and daft or large and unreachable it now seems. If it is a rainy, glum day when no inspi-ration flows, you can turn to your list for ideas. Make sure to include inexpensive treats, and those you can share with others. The following might give you some ideas:

> *have a day off – just play hooky and act spontaneously, seeing and doing just what you feel like when you feel like it*
> *have a bath to candle light*
> *go to the movies or a concert on your own*
> *take a long walk and explore a new part of your neighbourhood*
> *plan a day trip as far away as your budget will allow*
> *paint a wall in your favourite colour*
> *go to a dance class*
> *have a massage*
> *buy yourself a bunch of flowers or a flowering plant*
> *have a home facial – make a face mask from honey and eggs, and tone with cucumber juice*
> *book a reflexology session*
> *buy yourself a book of poetry, or borrow one from the library*
> *visit a gym for a fitness assessment, and steam or sauna afterwards*
> *buy a new costume and go swimming*

WORKING FOR CHANGE

You have instigated profound changes in your life, and you can use change itself to reinforce your intention and make following things through even easier. Most of what we do is habit-bound. We will usually have our own personal routines and timetables, as well as our very own individual way of doing things. This is true right down to the minutae of our everyday lives. Notice this for yourself next time you brush your teeth – you will probably always do exactly it in precisely the same way. There is tremendous comfort to be found in routine, and when we perform tasks and activities in the exact same way, it enables part of our brain to switch off from constant involvement and become involved in other things.

When we change one aspect of our lives, it can be stimulating and exciting, but big changes that run through every moment of our day can be very challenging. When you omit one element from a familiar task, your brain sends off alarm signals to remind you to include it. When these are ignored, you may notice yourself becoming uncomfortable because your mind knows that something is different. Sometimes the cravings that we have for things are not physically generated, but are a result of the mind working to remind us that our usual pattern has been broken.

There are two very important things to do in order to ease this. Firstly, we have to make sure that the message about our new resolve has been heard and received at every level of our being. This means re-educating ourselves about what we are doing and why, and also means using reminders to reinforce our intention. When you resolve to make a significant change, take some time to think it through. Rehearse the practical situations you will encounter, and play them in your mind's eye. This will let you anticipate how best you can achieve your desired change. See what it is like to do things in the new way – picture yourself waking through a whole day in your life; interacting with all the people you usually deal with, meeting all your commitments, as well as allowing some room for chance encounters and everyday happenings. See the new ways that you could do things, how easy and simple it is, and above all enjoy the experience.

Every time you do this imagining, you make a template in your mind. You can then return to it for reference if you are unsure about how to go about something, or if you are feeling uncomfortable. You are developing a store of memories that your mind can refer to if you feel unsure about what is going on. This can be tremendously useful during times of change, and every minute you spend imaging yourself responding differently or in your new way within familiar situations, really does pay off. You will soon find that situations where you have spent time imaging are actually significantly easier to deal with and more fruitful.

Use whatever personal time you can to reinforce your intention, and take it deep into your awareness. When you relax, take the message of your current change right down inside yourself by repeating it with every breath you take. Hear an inner voice speak those few words in a relaxed, calm and authoritative manner, and repeat them in exactly the same way over and over again. Feel yourself being hypnotised by the message, and by the gentle lilting tone you hear. Make your message succinct, and extremely positive. Forget about 'trying to' or 'wanting to', 'having to' or 'needing to'. Good suggestions include: 'I no longer...' and 'I have become a...'. These messages are short and precise, and easy for your inner self to understand.

Remind yourself of your intended change in as many ways as you can. Programme your computer to flash an occasional message of support, or place notes where you will see them, to remind you of how well you are doing. Other ways to reinforce this message include the use of affirmations and rhyme.

AFFIRMATIONS

This is a marvellous way to short-cut your every day mental activity, and introduce new ideas for change. Take a short, simple statement with an easy rhythm, that encapsulates the specific change you desire. 'Today's the day I...' is good, or 'Now is the time for...'. 'Every day in every way I am getting better and better' is a familiar affirmation, but one that is rather more all-embracing than would be useful right now. The more precise you can be, the easier it will be to concentrate your energy on achieving that goal.

Repeat your affirmation to yourself whenever you have a spare moment. Repeat it in clusters of 25 repetitions, or just keep repeating it for as long a time as you have. This is great to do whilst walking or doing other routine tasks like sweeping leaves, or photocopying. You can say it out loud, or just hear it in your head. Whenever you get the opportunity, write down your affirmation. Again, repeat it in groups of 25 repetitions. Every time you see the message, hear the message, and speak the message, you reinforce the idea for yourself; strengthening it and firmly establishing it as part of your reality.

As well as choosing some messages to forward your intentions, affirmations can also be especially useful in a more general, esteem-building and supportive way. Consider adding an affirmation that is guaranteed to make you feel better about yourself, such as 'I am enough, I have enough, I do enough', or one that addresses your own personal concerns.

Using rhyme is a powerful way to encourage your mind to adopt the idea more fully. You can notice for yourself how some rhymes and rhythms (like those used in ads and ditties) remain happily in your mind for a long time. So happily, in fact, that it can often prove difficult to rid ourselves of crafty pieces of advertising. Make your own, and you harness the power of your mind to work for you in furthering your goal.

Choose simple rhymes with a few words that really drive the message home. Take your time to make sure that you get it absolutely right, have fun with it and then try it out a few times, noticing if there are any words that you need to change. Sometimes you can hit on the right 'inner slogan' straight away, other times it will change and develop as you refine your thoughts. Let your mind be filled with your clever, rhythmic reminder whenever you can.

PHYSICAL CHANGE

The second way to reinforce your desired change and make it easier on yourself, is to lose the reminders of your old habit. You need to programme your environment so that things outside of yourself support and reinforce your positive choices. You have the power to change everything about the way you lived your life, right down to the tiniest detail. Doing this for just one day will dislodge all the links you have forged between everyday activities and habits that now no longer serve you. This is a challenging and exciting technique that you can use as much as you feel able to. You may simply change a few key areas of your routine, or your life, or you can go for broke and overhaul your entire day.

Consider sleeping with your head at the other end of the bed. Set your alarm for half an hour earlier than usual. Do not take a shower, or take a bath instead. Change your morning routine as much as you possibly can, including sitting in a different chair to have your breakfast, and listening to a different radio programme. Walk rather than ride to work, or take a different route altogether. Use different entrances and take the lift if you usually climb the stairs. Buy a different paper, go somewhere else for lunch, and eat different things.

(If you are following the diet you will probably be doing this already.)

If you usually go to the pub in the evening, try going to see a film instead. If you would go to a friend's house, have them come to you instead, or both go out. If you are staying in to watch television, choose a different channel, listen to music, or read a book instead.

If you tend to spend every evening in, go out. Find a hobby or leisure pursuit, join a gym, a class or group, or start one. Remember the power that meeting new people holds, as it instigates change and can encourage new ways of being. If it seems that there is no possibility for change, do not forget that even the smallest things can have a marked effect – sit facing a different direction, or doing things in a different sequence and at a new time.

Change everything that you possibly can. This is rather like throwing a pack of cards up in the air, and watching to see where they will fall. If you put your energy and enthusiasm into creating a positive force for change in your life, then it can achieve quite spectacular results. Having addressed one major habit, you may find that other areas of your life will also benefit from change, and you might as well gather the momentum and do it now.

MANAGING STRESS

Learning to relax is one of the best tools you can use against stress. This, combined with diet, will mean that you are able to combat rising stress levels and deal with the long term effects of existing stress. Learning to relax is just like any other skill – it can take time and practice, but the process is very enjoyable!

It is empowering to be able to relax into the knowledge that you have taken a profoundly beneficial step towards enhancing your health, and that everything you do from now on can augment that. It might also be encouraging to look at things in a wider perspective – you know that although your own feelings are specific to you, you are not alone in them. Many people have been through their own battles with habits and addictions, and have won through. On a greater level, there is a host of external stimuli that will be influencing your actions right now, including the moon whose cyclic movements govern the flow of water through your body, your surges of energy and patterns of addiction. Just as the moon's cycle changes throughout the month, so our feelings and physical sensations can rise and fall. Uniting yourself in some way with the larger patterns of the Universe can help you realise that whatever you are feeling at this moment is part of a cycle, and that it will change and you will move on.

Surrendering yourself to a higher power, acknowledging your own self, accepting the force of love in your life and letting your god or gods in, are all ways that can enable you to ease the internal pressure of keeping going and getting it right. Sometimes it can feel as though you have to do it all, and when the work is tough, this can be daunting. Relax and let something greater than yourself take some of the pressure off, in whatever you feel you can.

Most of us are not able to relax 'naturally'. Rather, we need to learn or to remind ourselves how to do it. Stop for a moment every now and again throughout the day, and notice if your shoulders are hunched up, or if you are locked in a tight mental process of repetitive thoughts. Notice what happens when you feel overwhelmed by an impulse or an urge, and see how your body and mind tighten up. Combat these in an instant with a relaxation formula: Stop, take a a deep, cleansing breath and realise where you are right now.

Relaxation exercises will help you relax your body, and open your mind and your heart to experience wonderful feelings. You can build anchors into your relaxation exercises that you will be able to use if you face a stressful situation. These are small but potent reminders of the way your body felt when it was completely relaxed, safe and secure in your own energy. You can then employ these to reawaken soothing, capable memories when you feel you are in need of them. Over time, regular relaxation will render you less susceptible to stress and more able to cope with pressures and demands as they arise.

Meditation is another way to manage stress. This is like relaxation for your whole being – body, mind and spirit – and is a skill that can be learned. Meditation practice will quite naturally relax your physical body, and help your mind switch off. It also engenders tremendous feelings of peace, calm and a sense of being in touch with what really matters – a useful skill in managing stressful situations. One of the major benefits of meditation is how it enables us to learn about choice. When you are sitting peacefully, with a clear mind, thoughts will enter and try to occupy your time, and you develop your 'choice muscle' as you either concentrate on them, or let them pass by. When you are experienced at being in this place, where you can let ideas and notions pass you by however seductive they may be, you will find that skill is very much alive in your everyday life too.

Take some time every day to learn these skills if they are new to you, or to remember them if you have practised them before. Initially, take about 20 minutes to do any of the relaxation techniques on the next pages, or one of your own choosing. Practise at any time of day when you will not be disturbed, and make sure that the door is closed, the phone will not ring, etc. When meditating, again choose a quiet time, perhaps at the start of the day or at dusk, and allow yourself 20 minutes to start with. There are some meditation practices on the next few pages, or you may know your own. It is really very simple. Keep your practice regular throughout this month, sticking to the same time of day if you can, but making sure you come back to the exercises every day.

RELAXATION SKILLS

PHYSICAL RELAXATION

Take off your shoes and loosen your belt or any tight clothes. Lie on your back on the floor or another flat surface and close your eyes. Let yourself relax and take a few long, cleansing breaths. Make each in-breath as deep and full as you can, and when you breathe out, imagine any tension or tightness being carried out of your body with your breath. Become aware, while you are breathing, of the way your body is starting to feel a little heavier, and notice the support that you are receiving on the back of your head, down your spine, and beneath your arms and legs. Continue to breathe deeply, and release any unwanted tension so that it can be carried away every time you breathe out.

You may feel yourself starting to sink down as your postural muscles relax and allow yourself to be supported. Keep breathing, and when your out-breath feels as clear as your in-breath, slow your breathing a little and enjoy the sensations in your body. Keep breathing slowly and deeply for as long as you feel inclined to.

When you are ready to stop this exercise, open your eyes, and stretch your arms and your legs before slowly rolling over onto your side and resting there for a few minutes before you get up.

If you are introducing an anchor to this exercise, wait until you are fully relaxed and at the point where your out-breath is as clear as your in-breath, and you have no more tensions to release or let go of. At this point, make your anchor.

MAKING AN ANCHOR

This involves choosing an activity that you will be able to use later to remind you of what you felt like when you were totally calm and fully relaxed; safe and secure in your own energy. The easiest ones are: Touch your left wrist with your right hand; touch your fingers together; touch your nose with your finger; gently pinch the end of your little finger. These can all be done freely in public without anyone knowing what you are doing. Whichever anchor you have chosen, do it now, just once. That is all you need to do. Think that you are establishing a physical reminder, do it, and then continue your relaxation.

It usually takes 3-5 repeats before your anchor will be effective. Repeat it every time you do the exercise, and by the time you need to use it in another situation, it will be ready. Each time you use it, you strengthen and reinforce it, so be sure to incorporate it every time you relax.

To use your anchor, whatever situation you are in, take a breath and perform the physical movement or touch. That will be enough to let your body fully remember its feelings of safety, calm, restfulness and relaxation, and it will replicate them. Your body is a marvellous thing.

FULL BODY RELAXATION

This is a wonderful exercise to aid sleep, or it can be done first thing in the morning, or at any other time. However, it is deeply relaxing and likely to send you off to sleep, so be prepared and make sure that you allow plenty of time for it.

Lie on your back and make yourself comfortable. Close your eyes, and begin to relax. Keep your breathing deep, full and easy, and feel your body beginning to get heavier as you start to let go and completely relax. Take in deep breaths and as you breathe out, say the word 'relax' in your mind. Repeat this a number of times so that you can establish the idea firmly.

You are going to cover your entire body, beginning with your toes and ending with your head, moving from one area to the next in a clear, gentle sequence – relaxing every bone, muscle and joint as you go. Start with your next in-breath, and picture your little toe on your left foot. As you breathe out and say the word 'relax' in your mind, see your little toe change as it relaxes. You might see it lengthen slightly, or become softer and fuller. You might see yourself turning off the lights there, and letting that part sleep. Whatever your image, breathe in, see that part, and as you breathe out watch it change as you say the word 'relax' silently to yourself. Move from your little toe to the next toe, then the middle one, and so on – from the ball of your left foot to the arch, then the heel. Relax your ankle your shin and calf, your knee joint, thigh and hip, before moving on to your right leg, and starting with the little toe there.

Take your time with this, there is no race. It will usually only take one breath to relax a spot. However a larger area, like a thigh, might require a few breaths, perhaps while you relax the front, then the back, the outside, and then the inside. If you know your anatomy, you can relax each muscle in turn, otherwise be guided by area.

When your whole body has been relaxed, if you are awake, take a few long, cleansing breaths and enjoy the feeling of this deep, comfortable relaxation. If you are introducing an anchor, do that now. Follow the directions in the first relaxation technique. When you are ready, slowly open your eyes, and then stretch out your arms and legs. Take a deep breath, and stretch again. Roll over on to your side, and rest for a few minutes before getting up.

WIDE AWAKE RELAXATION

When your body relaxes, certain identifiable things happen to your muscles, and you start to feel definite sensations like warmth and ease. Replicating these is a useful exercise for your mind, and some people find it extremely effective. It is a good technique if you find it hard to switch off your mind, or if you have an active imagination that you want to use.

Loosen any tight clothes, sit or lie down in comfort and close your eyes. Take a few deep, relaxing breaths to settle yourself, and release any obvious tensions. Now imagine your left arm beginning to feel very slightly warmer, heavier, and fuller than it was. Take your time to really feel these sensations. Notice how your arm seems to expand slightly, or become softer. Enjoy the sensation of warmth as it spreads though the limb right down to your finger tips. Now, encourage your right arm to follow suit. Maintain your sense of deep relaxation in the left arm, and encourage your body to balance itself, making both arms feel relaxed.

Move on through the rest of your body, until you are completely relaxed and comfortable. Register this feeling consciously – ask your mind to remember just what it feels like so that you can return to this feeling whenever you need to. If you are introducing an anchor, this is the time to do it. The instructions are in the physical relaxation technique on the previous page. Otherwise, simply luxuriate in the warm feeling of comfort and deep ease, and enjoy it. When you are ready, take a few deep breaths and then open your eyes. Breathe deeply for a minute or two, and then stretch out your legs and your arms, feeling the stretch right down to your toes, and out to your finger tips. Repeat the stretch, and remain still for a moment or two before getting up.

ACTIVE RELAXATION

This involves you actively identifying each part of your body in turn, so that you can be sure to relax it. It is a good exercise if you are feeling out of touch with your body, or have any anxiety about your ability to relax and let go.

Begin by sitting or lying comfortably. Take off your shoes, and loosen any tight clothing. This exercise is easily done in a chair, but if you feel more comfortable lying down, that is fine too. Close your eyes, and take a few deep breaths to relax and calm you. Let your breathing deepen and find its own natural and continuous easy rhythm. You are going to physically tighten, and then relax all your muscle groups, one after another until your whole body has been tensed and then relaxed, starting with your toes and moving up to your scalp.

Start with your left foot. Breathe in and tense the muscles in your left foot – really curl up the toes and hold the muscles tight. Breathe out and feel the tension mounting as you squeeze those muscles. The next time you breathe in stop for an instant at the top of your breath, and then as you breathe out, let go. Let the muscles in your foot relax completely and let your foot simply drop, heavy, fuller and warmer than before. With your next breath in and out, just appreciate that feeling, and notice the good sensations in your foot. Take another breath to do that too if you like. When you are ready to move on, clench the muscles in your right foot, and repeat the process. Give yourself time to fully appreciate the good sensations, and then move on – to your left calf, then your right, your left knee, then your right, etc. Continue up your body relaxing every area you can identify, including your face and your scalp. When you reach the top, scan your body and see if there are any areas that you missed, or that still hold some residual tension and return there to repeat the process.

When you are finished, just stay still and enjoy the experience. Let your mind relish the silence. If you are introducing an anchor, do that now. (The directions are with the physical relaxation exercise on the previous pages.) Continue to breathe deeply and take as long as you want before opening your eyes. Stretch out your arms and legs a few times and then take a minute more before getting up.

MEDITATIONS

Meditation is conventionally practised while sitting very still, but there are also dynamic forms that involve careful relaxed movements, and it is possible to do everything in your life in a meditative way. You might, for instance, make preparing a meal a meditation. Think just of Zen simplicity, and be silent, concentrating on every movement you make, action by action. Breathe in and out deeply, and be slow and careful as you choose, sort and chop. Consider nothing else except what you are doing in the moment. Honour the spirit of the ingredients you are preparing, and treat them with respect. Forget any notions you have about cutting carrots a certain way, and let the spirit of the dish guide your hands. Stir love into your cooking bowl. Fully embody your role as powerful co-creator in making ready the nourishment that you need for ongoing health and well-being.

Meditation has been described as a way of finding inner peace, or of connecting with the Universe. It is an extremely simple thing to do that contains a great elegance. It is a way of finding and staying in touch with the central, constant core of who you are – irrespective of emotions that are swimming around, what frame of mind you are in, or your physical shape. It is akin to discovering a lush oasis at the centre of your being, and knowing that you will be able to return there to rest, replenish, and enjoy discovery whenever you choose.

To meditate, you will need to set aside some time when you will not be disturbed by the outside world, and make yourself comfortable. Take off your shoes and sit comfortably with your back straight and your legs crossed, or with your feet flat on the floor if you are sitting on a chair. Then, close your eyes and do nothing – which for some people is extremely difficult. You need to not get caught up in your thoughts or to let them carry you away. Instead, find a position within yourself from which you can watch your thoughts pass by. Some of them will interest you, some may surprise you, and initially, all of them will seem very seductive. Your usual habit of responding to interesting thoughts is to follow them, and meditation is about learning a new way to interact with your mind's work.

One good technique when introducing yourself to meditation, is to be very aware of what is going on for a short while, so that you are supremely conscious of all the things that might crop in and disturb you. Begin by closing your eyes and scanning the area around you with your senses. Be clear about all the noise you can hear – the gentle hum of electricity passing through the room; traffic in the distance; birds singing nearby. Then consider all the aromas you can smell – the leather of your shoes; damp earth outside the window; your lover's perfume.

Register all of these impressions, and know that they are real, and there, and a part of your world. Work through all your senses – what do you see on the screen in your mind's eye; what can you taste on your tongue, and what can you feel? Be aware of the smallest stimulus like the lingering peppermint of your toothpaste, the cool cotton cloth of your clothes, the movement of the air you are breathing as it touches the skin on your face around your nose and upper lip. When you have registered all these impressions, what else is there? Try not to think an answer, but just sit and let it wash over you, until it is time to get up.

Other techniques that you might like to try include staring at a sharp image – perhaps a brightly coloured shape from a piece of card – and then closing your eyes and retaining that image in your mind's eye, so that you have something to focus your attention on. Candle flames are also good for this, and you can use the time you spend staring at the candle flame to relax yourself before you begin your meditation. Some people find the use of a mantra guides and settles them. This is just a word or a short phrase that has special meaning and that, again, gives the mind something on which to focus. You might know your own word, or might consider: Peace, Calm, or Love.

One of my favourite meditation techniques is humming. You sit, relaxed, and ready to start; your meditation is to hum for 20 minutes. There is no right way, or special breathing involved – you just breathe in, and when you breathe out you hum each time. At the start this may seem odd, but there will come a point where you stop consciously humming, where you no longer need to concentrate on it, but it just seems to happen. You no longer know if you are humming, or hearing humming, or being hummed. It is a magical, transformative experience that is uniquely different each time, and to each person.

Placing yourself in the tranquillity and the scattered order of nature is one of the most destressing things you can ever do. Being close to any body of moving water will soothe and cool you, and you can picture any cares being carried away from you. The asymmetry and casual form of the shapes, and the rich blend of colours in the natural world all have a restful and rejuvenative effect on your system. Simply gazing at a natural landscape full of rounded, uneven shapes in gentle shades of intrinsic colour will settle you. Seeing the irregularity of nature, such as still water by rocky mountains, will help you to gain a perspective on the essential rough and smooth quality that life itself holds. Exercising, relaxing, eating and meditating in the open air will all benefit your health, increasing your exposure to sunlight, your oxygen uptake and your sensory input.

Regular meditation practice, of whatever type you choose, will aid relaxation, improve your body's ability to heal and repair itself, and increase your own inner strength. This will show physically as your skin begins to glow. Practice meditating every day throughout the month of this diet, and then reassess how you are feeling within yourself.

FUELLING THE FIRE

For the time in your life when you did it, smoking was a powerful thing. You were instrumental in a strangely magical, alchemical process that proved your mastery over that which was stolen from the gods – the element of fire. It was present in every aspect of your life.

Now you have taken your life into another phase and the way you handle power and interact with the sacred in your life will change. Before, when you felt vulnerable in a relationship you could erect an actual smoke screen to avoid intimacy, or to make yourself feel protected. When you were in a situation in which you needed time to think, you had a physical activity that would gain you time in a socially acceptable way. Perhaps you would use the smoke if you were bored, or to quell desires and hungers within you. Now you will be addressing those feelings and finding other strategies for coping, but smoke and fire can still be present in your life in a number of special ways.

The sun is the primary element of fire in all our lives. Beyond ensuring life on the planet, it has a vital role to play in our ongoing health, yet we rarely pay it much attention. When the sun's rays touch the skin they promote the health-giving actions of Vitamin D and E, and the sun's light has important implications for mental and emotional health. Many types of minor depression can be resolved with regular and adequate amounts of sunlight. Light boxes are available that will simulate the sun's light and brighten up even the longest winters, but there are few days so overcast that spending an hour outdoors will not have a similar effect. Such exposure to sunlight will also work to regulate the body's cycles. However, the planet's protective layers have been so damaged that it is vital to make sure that your daily prescription is for sun light rather than burning, and care needs to be taken to avoid too much exposure when the sun's rays could cause harm. Early morning and late afternoon are good times.

When the sun is at it's highest point in the sky above us each day, our own digestive fire is also at its peak. This is the best time of day to plan your main meal so that the foods you eat will be burned up most efficiently and quickly.

Smoke is seen as a reminder of the world of Spirit. When material things burn, they transform into something ephemeral – changed yet still present, manifesting the qualities of air rather than form. Incense has long been used to represent Spirit and the transformational nature of our own lives. Modern religious ceremonies often include incense and this can add enormously to the atmosphere and meaning of the services. Our ancient forbears used fire to represent the greatest alchemical magic that changes all it meets and leaves nothing untouched. Modern associations also include the fire of our own feelings and physical passions, and the intensity of our dreams and desires.

Shamans and many traditional peoples burn a mix of special herbs to signify a change from everyday awareness into non-ordinary reality or dream time, and they are also used to cleanse an area. You can buy a mixture of these cleansing herbs, or those that will attract a blessing, either loose or in 'smudge' sticks. These are loosely tied thick bundles of herbs, including sage, that can be burnt and used to spread the cleansing smoke by hand. Consider cleansing your home energetically by using one of these smudging herbs, and let the positive smoke work to fill your own personal space with all that you hope and wish for yourself. Alternatively, burn some incense or joss sticks to accompany your relaxation or meditation. These will perfume your surroundings, influence your emotional and physical well-being, and augment your awareness of Spirit. Choose woody scents and varieties like sandalwood and amber for their smoky, resinous essence.

You can burn bunches of herbs that you have dried and bound yourself – choose rosemary, sage and lemon balm which are all very easy to grow in a pot on a light windowsill if you do not have space in a garden. They give off a woody, dry smell. The smoke from the smudge bundles is usually profuse and will leave a lingering, heavy scent, so make sure it is one that you like.

Essential oils extracted from woods and plants can also be burned in the house to fragrance an area and utilise fire and smoke in a smaller way. Choose from the wide variety of pure aromatherapy oils, and consider sandalwood, howood, amber, thyme, olibanum and rosemary.

Fire itself can represent the joy and laughter that bring a spark to your life. Laughter actually has a number of specific health benefits, so being happy and enjoying your life is important! When you smile, the way your facial muscles are pulled exerts a tiny but significant pressure on the area of your brain that is responsible for good feelings, and encourages it to release endorphins needed for your body to continue that response. Laughing frees your diaphragm and facilitates deeper, easier breaths. It also triggers the presence of an important immune response that will help fight airborne germs and protect you from colds and flu.

Be sure to seek out situations, activities and people to spark your enthusiasm and keep your inner fire well stoked. Enthusiastic socialising can burn as many calories as some exercise, and will also raise your metabolism. This is the efficiency of your body's ability to burn up the food you eat and release energy from it. The better your metabolic rate, the more effective you are at getting energy when you need it, and the less likely you are to store fat.

Taking regular exercise is a very good way of keeping your metabolism working at an optimum, and now you have the opportunity to introduce yourself to a more active lifestyle. Exercise does not have to be a formal event; you can increase the levels of activity in your life and experience all the knock-on benefits quite easily. One of the most immediate and positive effects is that your circulation will be improved and you are less likely to feel the cold, especially in areas like your hands, feet and bottom.

Turning up the heating for a short time will enable you to relax into the feelings of warmth and comfort that surround you when fire is active in your life. If you have an open fire or access to a real flame, so much the better. Otherwise, you can enjoy bonfires, and bring fire safely indoors with wax candles. Their flame is as real as any other fire, and its containment makes it especially useful at this time because it is portable, and can be an important and private symbol for you. You can use your candles to replace electric lights for a short time, or place extra ones on your mantlepiece, or altar if you have one. Bathe by candle light for a deliciously restful and sensual treat, and light one on your bedside table to relax you as you wind down and prepare for sleep.

You can reflect fire in the colours you choose to have around you in your home and in the rest of your life. Colours all have meanings because they influence many different aspects of our selves, stimulating or relaxing our energy and strengthening or releasing feelings. Red is a strong energiser, and even a touch of it will go a long way. Keep a Ponsettia plant or the Easter Cactus. Simply adding a piece of red ribbon or cord will be enough to energise and draw your attention to an aspect of your life. Fix it to the edge of your work desk to enliven it, or tie it around a plant pot. Yellow is a strengthening and uplifting colour that can remind you of the sustaining warmth of the sun. This is a wonderful colour to use in the kitchen, or where you will be eating, because of its strong associations with digestion.

Extend the range of firey colours to include pink. This uplifting and joyful colour is reputed to represent the emotions, and to encourage the heart. Consider planting a Fuschia or a Busy Lizzie, or keeping something pink near your bed. A fresh coat of paint, or even a flame coloured scarf, or a brightly covered notebook are economical ways to reinforce this. Choosing bright red, yellow and orange foods – and cooking and serving dishes – will bring fire into your kitchen. Make menu choices of carrot soup, roast pumpkin and squashes, and peach chutney. Cooking on a real flame is a wonderful way to achieve this energy too, and the odd meal made on a camping stove can bring fire to life.

Changes to your physiology will effect the way your muscles

work, and now is a good time to treat yourself to some body therapy that will both relieve any aches and pains (see Massage, page 31) and work to redress and re-educate any postural difficulties. A visit to your osteopath might be in order, but you can also work yourself to reassess your posture and rediscover how best to be comfortable in your new body with your new habits and ways.

You can ease your posture in an instant by raising your sternum or breastbone up out of your waist, and loosening your neck. Imagine that there is a fine, strong thread hooked on to the ceiling just above and in front of your head. The other end attaches to a point on the centre of your breastbone. Aim to keep an exquisite tension in this thread, and enjoy the greater lung capacity and relief from muscle tension that instantly follows as your chest is lifted and your shoulders relax back.

Release any congestion in your neck by relaxing your jaw and letting your chin carry your head back slightly. Picture your spine lengthening as you do this, and feel your head balancing loosely on the top of your spine. Let it 'wobble' from side to side a little to see just how freely and loosely it moves when there is no restriction. Use these techniques whenever you remember through the day, and soon the postures will become easier and more usual for your body.

You may find that some old familiar aches and pains disappear as toxins are flushed out of your system and your nervous system begins to send more relaxed messages to your muscles. Your breathing pattern will also be different, and your diaphragm will be working more effectively, changing the way your shoulders sit, and easing tension in your neck. Try the following postural exercises to relieve any residual holding patterns and re-educate your body.

The most common sites of tension are the stomach, bottom, and the neck and shoulder area. This sequence of exercises can be repeated every day, and will flow into a smooth and relaxing routine, or you may find one is most suitable for you. Used over time, these exercises relax, strengthen and re-educate important groups of postural muscles that can have a significant impact on how you feel.

TUMMY TENSER

Get into a comfortable position on your hands and knees on the floor, with your hands just below your shoulders, and your knees evenly spaced. Keep your shins flat on the floor straight out behind your knees. Look down at the floor just in front of you, and take a few deep, relaxing breaths. Relax your shoulders. Then suck in your tummy as far as you can, aiming to touch your spine with your belly button. Pull it in as far as you can, letting your lower abdominal muscles pull up and in as they curl in your pelvis too. Hold this for three breaths, then release, and repeat three times.

This is an excellent exercise for toning the abdominal muscles, and works very well to help you identify these muscles so that you can hold them, and relax them, whenever you remember.

BOTTOM BUSTER

Stand easily, with your arms hanging loosely by your sides and your feet about shoulder width apart. Take a few deep, relaxing breaths. Now pull in your lower abdominal muscles and at the same time pull up with your gluteus. These are the muscles that cover your bottom. Imagine you are trying to stifle a loss of air and hold them tight, so that you are pulling up the whole region. Hold for three breaths, then release them and take two or three deep, relaxing breaths. Repeat three times.

This is remarkably effective for toning up the whole bottom area, and also enables you to identify and relax the muscles if tense.

SHOULDER ROLL

Sit with your back straight and your feet flat on the floor. Relax your shoulders and take a deep breath. Lift and rotate your right shoulder to make an imaginary circle in the air, and then do the same with your left shoulder to loosen up the main muscles in the area. Do this a few times until your shoulders feel loose and your arms are hanging freely. Then slowly roll your head forwards until your chin is touching on to your chest. Take a few deep breaths and let your neck relax further. Now put your hands on your head and feel their weight pulling down on your neck, stretching it just a little further. Do not pull down on your head, just relax your arms and let them draw your neck into a greater stretch. Keep breathing, and notice how your head descends a little with each deep out-breath that you make. Take your time with this, and let yourself take at least 6-8 deep, easy, relaxed breaths. Then lift your arms up and put them back down by your side, and slowly and carefully straighten up your neck until you are looking forwards in front of you again. Now let your chin drop loose so that your mouth opens, and pull your head back slightly on your neck. Feel the slight tension at the back of your head, and then take another deep breath.

This works to loosen the whole neck and shoulders area, and is a remarkably effective treat that can be repeated whenever tension starts to build.

STAYING WARM

It is very important to keep physically warm. Fluctuating energy levels throughout this period of transition mean that your temperature is likely to be less constant. It might be a new habit for you to attend to your body like this, but it is valuable in conserving and redistributing your own inner elemental fire. Make sure that you wear an extra layer for at least the next month, and keep your head, hands and feet warm. This is especially relevant if you are sitting down all through an evening, or have a sedentary job. Women will also want to ensure that their legs and feet stay warm from mid-cycle and ovulation right through to the period. That just means keeping socks or slippers on and minimising barefoot experiences until the warm weather returns. Instigate regular comfort checks for yourself. Take just a second to check through your own list of potential tension spots and discomforts, using your attention to review what is happening in your body.

- Make sure you are breathing! Seriously, it is very common to hold your breath.
- Are you warm enough/not too warm?
- Are you relaxed – where is the tension being held in your body? Are your·toes curled or is your jaw clenched? Check your own

familiar tension spots.

Make this an automatic review that you repeat every hour for a few days until you get used to the way you feel and are able to stay within your own comfort zone.

FINDING THE CENTRE

Staying comfortable in your body is much easier if you have developed your own inner physical sense of your self. Feelings of being centred or grounded will help you keep your body as a focus for your own well being.

CENTERING YOURSELF

Close your eyes for a moment. Where are you? Where is the spot that you perceive to be the centre of yourself, the place where your awareness rests when you are not consciously aware of it? You may find it is in some unpredictable place like in between your eyes, or three inches in front of your head. Relax and take a few easy, deep breaths, and imagine yourself breathing directly into this centre while you gently and carefully draw it in and down your body, relocating it in a special place just below your belly button. Move slowly and respectfully with it, stopping if you encounter any resistance, but otherwise continue until you feel quite settled. You will notice marked changes as you do this. Your breathing will deepen and become slightly smoother and easier, and you may well feel a little warmer and experience a sense of strength and security.

Once you have settled, place your hands over that spot, letting them rest there while you take a few more full, relaxed breaths, and luxuriate in the experience.

Every time you do this it reinforces the new sensation of being permanently settled and centred securely within yourself. Once you get used to doing it, you will be able to refer to these feelings whenever you choose. Simply close your eyes and use your awareness to confirm how centred you are, then you can let your remembered experience guide you back.

GROUNDING

Use your imagination with each of these two lovely exercises to reinforce your physical feelings and senses. They are an object lesson in how intimately the mind and body work together.

DEVELOPING ROOTS

Stand with your feet about shoulder width apart and your arms hanging loosely by your sides. Keeping your weight evenly on both feet, start to sway gently backwards and forwards. Keep your movements small and simple, but rhythmic. Use your arms to augment the movements and let them swing. Enjoy the feelings and sensations of moving freely and easily, as if being moved by a soft and refreshing summer breeze. Feel the pleasure of moving your body through the air, while staying strongly and securely based in one place. Close your eyes to deepen the experience.

Now imagine your root system reaching down into the ground and anchoring you within the earth. Trace your roots as they run deep into the ground and fan out around the space you occupy. Notice how solid and established you feel and impress this on your mind to remember later. Stay for a while simply enjoying these sensations. When you are ready, become still again and open your eyes. Stand there for a few minutes to let your energy settle.

HOOKING UP

Sit with your eyes closed and take some deep, relaxing breaths Breathe right down to the base of your spine and notice how easily and well the rest of your spine balances on top of this point. Take your time and feel how comfortably your body fits together above this strong base. Return your awareness to that point at the very bottom of your back, and imagine that you have a tail – a beautifully elegant, long, swishy tail, and see it extend away from you and reach down into the floor beneath and just behind you. Stay with it as it stretches sleekly down into the soil below you, and travels on down into the ground, reaching on further and further through the earth. See it reaching into the very centre of the planet, and in the space that you find there; notice your own hook that is just perfect for your tail to wrap around and secure itself on to. Once you are sure that you are safely anchored, return your awareness to your body and enjoy the feeling of being fully at home and anchored here.

This is a great way to combat any 'spacer' tendencies, and you can do this very quickly whenever you need to feel secure and grounded in the world.

FOOD

Food is one of your most powerful healing tools, and the energetic qualities of your meals will have a tremendous impact on your overall health. There are some specific areas which you will be able to identify as being in need of attention, and food is an immediate and effective way to draw energy to where it is most needed. You will:

- Regulate blood sugar levels.
- Stabilise your weight and any energy fluctuations.
- Improve and maintain good elimination, and speed the expulsion of toxic residue from your system.
- Restore optimum vitamin and mineral levels.
- Reactivate your taste buds and your sense of smell.
- Restore health and vitality to all your body systems.
- Ensure adequate available energy for all your needs.

Part of your body will be wanting the security of familiar habits. However, it is crucial that you do not let yourself be seduced into continuing old patterns of eating that do not serve your best purpose right now. Make definite, positive choices for change, and stick with them.

Putting something in your mouth is a remarkably effective and fast-acting way of influencing your whole body. What your taste buds register soon becomes a system wide response, and its effects will influence your digestion as profoundly as any other measure. Now you have a chance to let your gut recover from the constant irritation caused by nicotine, and can gently warm and encourage peristalsis while you concentrate on your own positive nutrition.

Taste is one important consideration for a balanced approach to nutrition (see page 21) but foods also contain nutritional and medicinal properties. Balancing our need for a regular intake of protein, fat and carbohydrate is every bit as important as making sure we have foods that help us feel soothed and grounded, and that provide instant and accessible energy.

VITAMINS AND MINERALS

Right now, your body will need foods and supplements to address a range of nutritional deficiencies. There is an immediate need for Vitamin C to soothe and heal every part of your body, especially the immune system. Vitamin A will work to reinforce the mucus membranes and help the skin repair. The range of B-vitamins will address and calm a jangly nervous system and work to improve the quality of your sleep and the texture of your skin. Vitamin E will fight the internal effects of smoking and is essential to the health of your muscles, skin, and reproductive system. Among the minerals, Zinc, Chromium, Manganese, Magnesium, Boron, Calcium and Iodine will all have been compromised, and they will be needed to ensure a return to optimum health and vitality.

All vitamins, minerals and trace elements work together in the body to ensure full health, so a full range of nutrients is necessary to address any ongoing health concerns. Vitamins and minerals are present in the foods we eat, and the following table makes some suggestions for good food sources. Make sure you read the following piece about growth, storage and preparation and the way they can affect the presence of vitamins and minerals. Vitamins are easily damaged – Vitamin C for instance is destroyed by air, heat, light, metals and alkaline substances, so when you cut a fruit and expose it to the air, and when you cook it, you are losing the valuable vitamin.

VITAMINS:

VITAMIN A	all yellow fruits, flowers and vegetables – apricots, corn, carrots, squash and pumpkins, violet leaves, dandelion buds, papaya, watercress, mint, lettuce, chicory and dairy foods
VITAMINS B	all green vegetables especially broccoli, nuts and seeds, whole grains, eggs
VITAMIN C	all raw, fresh foods especially parsley, black currants, broccoli and other green vegetables, citrus fruit and potatoes
VITAMIN D	sunflower seeds, eggs, dairy produce
VITAMIN E	sunflower seeds, olives, coconuts and their oils
VITAMIN K	all dark green leafy vegetables, cauliflower, cabbage, carrot tapes, kale, soybeans, alfalfa, seaweed

MINERALS:

CALCIUM	kelp, nettles, parsley, chamomile flowers, oats, chicory, dandelion, watercress, seeds and nuts
CHROMIUM	black pepper
MAGNESIUM	nuts, figs, dates, soybeans, cowslips, dandelion, kelp, marshmallow, oats, parsley, raspberries, watercress, spinach
MANGANESE	nuts, all dark green leafy vegetables, beetroot, avocados, egg yolk, sunflower seeds, pineapple, kelp, whole grains
POTASSIUM	parsley, wheatgerm, dandelion leaves, bananas, apricots
SELENIUM	cereal and whole grains, nuts and fruit
ZINC	pumpkin and sunflower seeds, green leafy vegetables
IODINE	sea vegetables and seaweeds

OTHER FOOD ATTRIBUTES

There will also be other nutrient needs. It is vital, for example, to redress any imbalance in intestinal microbes, and foods such as live yoghurt can help with this. Reducing the sugar and yeast in your diet will also have a beneficial effect because this will starve off any bacteria that are less than useful.

If you are feeling the loss of stimulants, make sure you are having regular meals and giving your body enough energy to cope. Choose high energy foods that will meet all your needs. Raw foods, fruits and seeds are power houses of energy that will give the same sort of lift as sugary sweets and treats, but will be easier on your system and more healthful. Move beyond apples and think about the deliciousness of your favourite fruit, or an exotic medley of mango, pineapple and passion fruit, and the sensual pleasure of a sweet, juicy tangelo.

Other important considerations include stabilising energy fluctuations, and recognising the effects that individual fruit and vegetables have on your system. Hot flushes and occasional shivers are not uncommon at this time, and the careful choice of foods, herbs and spices can work to balance this. The colour of foods is a strong indicator as to their health-giving benefits. Yellow and orange foods are generally great for the spleen, being high in Vitamin A and betacarotenes (squash, pumpkin, corn, carrots, parsnips, etc.). These will work with the spleen to help keep the energy moving in your body, and will encourage you to settle back into regular biological cycles. Make sure you include some as often as possible.

Eat beetroot and bitter greens to give your liver a boost and reinforce its work as chief cleanser in the body. Take mung beans and whole grains to soothe digestion and enhance elimination, and eat plenty of fruit and vegetables for energy and their vital elements. Coriander is a wonderful cooking herb that will smooth out any digestive upsets, and both mung and soya in all its guises will help even out energy rushes. Fruit is easily digested and is gentle on the stomach. It is amongst the most cleansing and valuable of foods and will clear toxic residues from your system while supporting your body and maintaining energy levels. Fruit that is grown naturally, without chemicals, and is picked when ripe is the most healthful.

Mango is a rich source of Vitamins A and C, and works to soothe and regenerate the throat and the digestive system. Apples are particularly cleansing, and are especially useful for clearing muggy headaches and sinus congestion. Cherries ease pelvic congestion and generally stimulate the bowel. Pomegranates strengthen digestion and tonify the gut. Figs are an excellent tonic and reinforce pelvic health. Papaya relieves indigestion and clears and heals the g-i tract, as well as being one of the most delicious 'medicines' ever.

Grains are the most valuable foods in that their carbohydrate value provides energy and promotes the release of feel-good chemicals from the brain. They also provide fibre which reinforces vegetable fibre in maintaining the health of the gut. Whole grains also include B-vitamins, trace minerals and a small amount of protein.

Rice is useful for calming an irritated or inflamed gut. Whole grain rice has more B-vitamins, and can be a useful aid to relieving constipation, but basmati rice can be easier to digest. Barley is useful for dispelling fatigue and ridding the system of excess fluid. Rye and buckwheat are excellent for preventing the build up of fat in the system. Oats are warming and provide a slow, sustained release of energy.

Vegetables are rich in vitamins and are nourishing whilst being among the easiest foods to digest. Asparagus is a nerve and heart sedative and a mild laxative. Garlic is a powerful antibiotic, and the whole family have excellent cleansing qualities. Onions cleanse the system and soothe the gut. They are a wonderful remedy for piles. Okra is a useful anti-inflammatory that works well with cystitis, sorethroats, bronchitis and irritable bowel. Carrots purify the blood and strengthen the kidneys. Jerusalem artichokes are good for balancing blood sugar levels and are reputed aphrodisiacs.

Beans are low in fat, high in fibre, and provide protein, iron, B-vitamins and trace minerals. Aduki beans are a very good support for the kidneys. Mung beans are especially cleansing, and well tolerated by most digestions.

Herbs and spices work to activate healing functions in the body, as well as to please the palate and satisfy the taste buds. Cardamom calms and stimulates digestion. Ginger root whether fresh or dried adds warmth and zing to a meal, and will gently stimulate your appetite. Cinnamon warms and sweetens, and coriander cools, soothes, and enhances digestion. Fenugreek is a warming tonic. Saffron cools and tones the digestive system. Turmeric, the lovely powdered yellow root that adds colour and a hint of pungency to rice and curry dishes aids protein digestion and mobilises Vitamin C stores.

Many people associate the old habit with eating, e.g. having a cigarette in place of food, or to follow a meal. The *Just Quit!* diet allows the appetite to naturally re-assert itself. It also meets the need for strong tastes and flavours during the time when the taste buds are recovering and rediscovering their sensitivity. The focus is also on eating in a way to refresh and shake loose old habit patterns connected with mealtimes. If you are formulating your own dietary plans you will need to consider all these factors in working out your own best way forward. Look to the diet suggestions to schedule your meals too. The Moving On chapter at the end of this book includes some useful on-going dietary advice.

FOOD CHOICES

If you follow the *Just Quit!* diet for the next month, you will be able to decide which foods to eat from the lists that are given in each section of the diet. The foods have been carefully chosen to achieve the specific aims of each step of the diet. Common allergens like yeast and cow's dairy have been removed from the diet to make sure that your system is as settled as possible and safe from all aggravants.

Step 1 – Cleansing

This will cleanse your system of unwanted toxins, improve your body's elimination and meet all your energy needs. The fruits that you will find on this list are all high in natural sugars to provide you with the energy you need for your body to cleanse itself and to keep functioning well. They will also be easy to digest and not leave you feeling cold or heavy afterwards. When digestion is easy, and the food is warming, your digestive fire is easily able to cope.

Step 2 – Energising

Here your body can enjoy the slow release of energy from carbohydrates and regular mealtimes, in order to enable your adrenal glands to relax and settle into the comfort of consistently available energy. A regular intake of optimum nutrition is the best way to ensure ongoing energy levels while the body starts to rely on digestion rather than stimulants for its energy. Food choices here are carefully designed to ensure you do not experience energy slumps that can lead to cravings. You can follow your taste buds and choose between sweet and savoury, etc., and a full range of recipes supports your choices from the food lists.

Step 3 – Balancing and Revitalising

This consolidates the work of cleansing and energising, and restores a strong sense of well-being with a concerted approach to overall positive nutrition. Having made an excellent beginning with Steps 1 and 2, now you will be choosing foods that will ground you and continue to enhance elimination and improve digestion. They will support your ongoing maximum vitality, while consolidating the work of background cleansing and rejuvenation. This balanced eating plan will form the basis of your future health, and can become a springboard for ongoing well-being.

You can modify the length of each step to fit your own individual needs, or just take the structure and food choices, and develop your own ongoing eating plan.

THE NATURAL ORGANIC CHOICE

Wherever you can, choose food that is naturally or organically grown. The Soil Association mark is an absolute guarantee of quality and freedom from the plethora of herbicides, pesticides, treatments and other chemicals that are routinely used to grow most other foods. While you are ridding your body of poisons, it is a good idea not to introduce more! Organic choices are available at most supermarkets, and you may well have a local market where naturally-grown foods are sold, or a local organic grower's group.

When you choose a food that is grown chemically, you are robbing yourself of optimum nutrition. To stay within even UK government safety guidelines you will need to peel most fruit and vegetables before you eat them. As many of the nutrients are to be found in the thin layer just below the skin, you are throwing away much of the food's goodness. You will also be eating something that your body is going to have difficulty digesting, and you will be increasing the amount of detoxification and elimination your body will have to do to rid itself of the build up of chemicals in your system.

Nowadays, about 90% of your shopping can be organic or naturally grown – from herbs to grains – and although cost is a factor, it is worth spending more to ensure that as much of the food you are eating is really good for you. Genetically modified foods are regarded by many as a time bomb that could have phenomenal repercussions on our health, and even on the viability of our species. They are best avoided.

Most people would never dream of using a low grade petrol in their car. And you would never put any old disk into your computer, regardless of whether it might contain some form of virus or be about to damage or downgrade your software.

FRESH IS BEST

Fruit and vegetables start losing their nourishment the moment they are picked. The difference between truly fresh foods, and those we are used to buying from shops and stores, is enormous. Freshly picked peas really do taste sweet, and lettuces are not limp by nature! Most of us can manage to grow a few herbs or salad plants in pots on the window sill, in a window box, or a tub, and it is well worth doing so. It is one of the best ways to get vitamins and minerals, and will benefit your health enormously.

Foods you choose to buy need to be as fresh as possible to ensure that they are full of the nutrients you need, so reject any food that looks as though it has been stored for too long, and make sure that you eat it as soon as possible after purchase. It is better to shop little and often, buying small amounts of really fresh food each time. Store it well, refrigerating or handling gently, and be prepared to reject any foods that do not seem positively health giving. When the carrots and courgettes are soft and bendy, their nutrient level is very low, and you are cheating yourself if you eat them in that state. Choosing foods that are seasonally available ensures you will be eating them as fresh as possible, and therefore maximising the nutrients available to you.

Choose fresh, raw foods that have not been pre-prepared. Peeling and cutting into a fruit or vegetable breaks the cell walls and releases Vitamin C into the air, so it is lost to you. It is better to prepare them yourself – it does not take very long and the nutritional rewards are immense. Wherever possible choose fresh foods over tinned, canned or frozen.

Good food has its own natural flavour. It does not need to be chemically altered, pesticide laden, artificially flavoured, preserved, modified and added to. There is rarely any need for stimulants and flavour enhancers. All of these methods and additions do little to benefit our health, but much to ease and aid the profitability of food manufacture and production. When the spotlight is on restoring harmony and maximum health to your system, it is important to keep things as simple and healthful as possible.

When buying prepared foods, always read the labels. Check for added yeast and milk which tend to be added to a wide variety of foods, and screen out additives, preservatives, colourings and any foods that have only a number instead of a name.

ANIMALS

Some people do well on a diet that is rich in vegetable proteins, whereas other people benefit from eating meat in some form. Recent Dioxin, PCB, and CJD health scares in humans have all been traced back to the ingredients that animals have been fed. This routinely includes sweepings from the floors of the abbatoir, and sewage sludge! Unbelievably, these substances have been considered 'not deleterious' to their health, or to ours. Animals and their products, like milk, cheese, eggs and butter, raise moral issues beyond the health concerns associated with eating them. The way that most animals are farmed robs them and us of dignity, and treats them more like products to be manufactured than as sentient beings.

It is important that you make positive choices in this regard and if you are going to make meat a regular part of your diet, then it needs to have been organically reared and humanely killed. These are now available in many supermarkets and individual shops as well as by direct purchase from farms and cooperative shops.

EATING

The time you choose to eat is almost as important as what you choose, and will greatly affect your digestion. Stick to the timetables included in each step of the diet to give you a good framework for mealtimes, and then let your body's energy levels guide you. Eating breakfast is an absolute must, because you will not have had any energy in the form of food for maybe 12 hours. Your body will have been involved in replenishing itself, and will have been doing a lot of healing and repair work through the night. Making the switch into becoming physically and mentally active requires energy, and it is your duty to provide it – otherwise you are really asking your body to overtax itself. This is why you think you need a stimulant in the morning. Often you really just need some energy, and food is the best way to provide yourself with this. Similarly, do not eat a large meal just before going to bed, or you rob your body of the chance to digest it, and the opportunity for its overnight work of replenishment and rejuvenation. If you are not following the *Just Quit!* diet, then develop a structure to follow with regard to mealtimes, and stick to it for at least a month in order to balance your energy levels and then refine it to suit your ongoing needs.

How you eat is enormously important when you are working on enhancing your digestion and rebalancing your system. Be as relaxed as you can – never schedule business meetings for meal times, or try to have your meal while feeding others. Give yourself the gift of sitting down and enjoying your food. Taking food seriously means concentrating on the joy of meals to the exclusion of other distractions. If you focus on the food you are eating – how good it looks, the wonderful aroma and the delicious tastes, it is incredibly satisfying. This is much better than eating on the run, and simply feeding your face. Digestion starts in your mouth, so make sure you chew your food. This increases your enjoyment and feelings of satisfaction, will delight your taste buds, and leave you feeling as though you have eaten properly, rather than having bolted something down. It is important to infuse your mealtimes with a sense of relaxation so that your system can destress and focus on good nourishment.

Dedicate each meal to your own nourishment, physically and spiritually. Do this silently for yourself by inviting Spirit to partake of the meal, by taking just a moment to focus on your intention before you begin to eat, or by saying a blessing, prayer or 'Grace'.

Choose places where you can feel calm. Bright lights, primary colours, busy people coming and going and lots of noise do not enhance digestion, and will leave you wanting something else after you have eaten. Make mealtimes quiet and solitary or choose good, positive company that you enjoy.

It is essential to shake loose some of the habit patterns associated with meals, and Step 2 of the diet is specifically aimed at doing this. If you are not following the diet, make sure you alter your pattern of eating in as many ways as possible to ensure that it is a radically different experience, and one that will encourage you to attract and develop new health habits.

DRINKING

Make sure that what you drink is of the same quality as the foods you are eating. Choose good bottled water that comes in a glass bottle or that has been stored well out of direct light, or use a water filter – and drink lots of it. Sip slowly with a meal if you need to moisten your food, otherwise wait for a short time after eating and have a drink that will enhance your digestion. See page 91 for some choices. Do not drink anything cold or iced before eating. This is the certain to put out your digestive fire and make the meal harder to process. You will find recipe suggestions for drinks in each step of the *Just Quit!* diet.

The most important thing to remember about what, when and how you eat and drink, is that if you are not enjoying it, then you are missing out on the 'x factor' – the element that adds a phenomenal amount to the pleasure and effectiveness of your meal. Enjoy your meals, give yourself time and space in which to appreciate them, and have fun experimenting with the new tastes and flavours that you will be able to discern now that your taste buds have returned to normal.

THE DIET

The *Just Quit!* diet is presented in an easy-to-follow format that will guide you through each step. Before you embark upon Day 1, read through the lists of foods and drinks for that day, and the directions on preparation and when to eat them. Check the Timetable Notes for any special reminders. At the start of each step, read ahead for a few days to help you plan your shopping, and to ensure you are well prepared for all your dietary needs.

Do not undertake any part of the diet, or do any of the suggested support measures or exercises that you feel anxious about – that would defeat their purpose. If you have any medical concerns, or are under a practitioner's care, discuss this diet with them before you begin.

The diet is planned in three steps, but you can move forward or backtrack if you feel that one aspect of the diet is or would be most helpful. Be flexible, and use the diet plan as a loose structure if this is what will work best for you.

DAILY PLANS

TAKING A BREATH

Each morning when you wake up, before you do anything else, start one of the breathing exercises. Choose whichever one you like the most, or that you find easiest while you are lying down. Do the exercise before you get out of bed to make sure that your diaphragm is as relaxed and responsive as possible, and that you receive ample amounts of oxygen into your system before you are up and making demands of your body. Starting your day this way provides you with the energy that you need right from the start, and reminds your body what it feels like to be filled with fresh, clean air, and all the benefits that accompany that.

Expect to spend about five minutes working with your breath. If you find it very relaxing, and there is a risk of you going back to sleep, then set your alarm, or do your breathing exercise while sitting up in bed. Do not be tempted to skip this important step as it will set a breathing template for you to use throughout the day, and will establish a strong easy pattern of breathing that will help your body balance itself.

Once you are ready to get on with your day, you will need to wake up your taste buds. This is the first step to repairing and restoring full function to your digestive system.

WAKING UP YOUR TASTE BUDS

Your taste buds will have been in the front line of attack and will now be ready for transformation and re-educating. One of the main contributors to weight gain at this time is the desire of the taste buds to actually taste something! Strong, piquant flavours are a must to satisfy this need, and to stave off hunger pangs. Once your taste buds are satisfied, you will not want to eat more. Everybody has their own taste likes and dislikes, and there will be some flavours that you find you have more of an affinity with at certain times.

Early morning is one of the most difficult times whilst you are establishing change and balancing your energy levels. It is the ideal time to feed your taste buds, and let the experience awaken your entire system. Every morning, eat one of the foods or drinks from the list below. You can go back to the list once more during the day if you feel a wave of desire, and it will usually satisfy it. Take them soon after waking, before you have your breakfast, or drink anything, and try to vary your choice so that you do not always have the same thing. The first four items are the most successful in delivering a clear wake up call to your senses, but if you find them unpalatable, or something else appeals more, then follow your own inclination.

One of these needs to be taken every morning. Make sure you

have just a single piece, or a thumb-sized portion, or a small sip – these are not to satisfy a hunger, they are a surprise gift for your taste buds.

olives – choose green or black, stuffed with pimento or stoned
salted pistachio nuts
umeboshi plums
tonic water
strong goat's or sheep's cheese
fresh rocket, sorrel, or radiccio leaves

CLEANSING YOUR SYSTEM

Once your body is awake and you are moving around, have a hot drink from your daily list. This will encourage your body to cleanse itself of impurities that have built up during the night, and will give your kidneys a gentle flush. It will also gently warm your system, and prepare it for breakfast. Choosing neutral fluids at this time enables your body to wake up gently, and lets it respond to the temperature and nature of what you are taking. This is much kinder than giving it a strong hit of caffeine or other stimulant, and although it may take a little time to get used to, it means that your body will be able to wake itself up rather than having to rely on chemicals. By the end of this diet, you should find that you are waking up more easily, that your body is cleansing itself fully, and that you have good energy levels from the moment you wake up.

Once your system is used to waking up naturally, one of your first impulses will be to use the toilet. If your bowels are sluggish in the meantime, you might like to take your drink to the toilet with you, and just sit and sip – practised regularly this will soon encourage a regular bowel movement. Otherwise, take the time to sit and drink quietly, and consider what you will have for breakfast.

Decide for yourself what works best in your timetable – you may like to have breakfast first, and then head for the bathroom, or want to cleanse completely before sitting down to eat. Even if you are running late it is important to make time to start your day well.

Bathing Massage

Use your bath-time routine to add a little extra treat in your body care. Use your time under the shower or in the bath to carefully massage every part of your body with the moisturising suds of soap or gel. You have to cover all your body anyway, and this is a good way to express loving care that takes only a few seconds longer than normal. Make sure you have lots of suds on your hands, and use sweeping strokes over all your long bones, and small, round ones over each joint. Starting with your shoulders, make lengthy sweeps from your neck out, then cleanse around your shoulder joint and under your armpit, before sweeping down and up your upper arm, around your elbow, down and up your forearm, around your wrist, and so on. Use sweeping strokes over your torso, and then make a circular movement around your breasts and your hip joints. Carry on down to your toes, along your feet, and make small circles around the joint of each toe. When you are finished, every part of your body will feel as though it has been touched and lovingly woken up, ready for getting into fresh clothes and moving along with the day ahead.

Throughout the day, every drink will give you an opportunity to cleanse and refresh yourself, and each small cleansing action is an opportunity to rid yourself of physical toxins and to prepare yourself for the tasks ahead. Washing your hands can be a chance for another mini massage – hands are so often ignored, and will benefit if you wash carefully around the wrists, down the palm, around each joint and knuckle and make cleansing sweeps off each finger.

FUELLING YOUR BODY

Always have breakfast. Make your choice from the recommended foods on the daily list. Take the time to sit and relax and make sure you give yourself the energy that you will need for the day to be as easy and pleasant as possible. If you enjoy opening your mail, or doing the crossword, then you can do this as you eat. If you prefer, you can also make this meal a prayer, or a meditation. Breakfast may be the only meal of the day that you will have alone, and you can use the opportunity to really commune with your self.

Simply stop and consider what you are doing as you take in each mouthful and begin the wonderful process of transformation from whatever is on your plate to the fuel that will make your body work, move, function and achieve your goals. Savour each mouthful, and only take another when your mouth is empty. Chew well, and feel the goodness of each ingredient. Realise the importance of your food choices, and what a gift you are making to yourself – the gift of life. Notice the way your body feels when you are nourishing yourself well and let satisfaction expand your experience of eating.

Be sure to allow ample time for meals in your day. If you are eating with others, make a rule not to discuss work, and avoid business meetings – they rarely encourage good digestion. Eating with people whose company you enjoy can enrich the whole experience of the meal; enhancing nourishment on other levels too. If you are eating alone, still prioritise – close the office door, take the phone off the hook, switch off the television – let yourself be fully nourished by the foods you eat.

In Step 2 of the *Just Quit!* diet there are specific directions to ensure that your energy and blood sugar levels are kept constant. Otherwise, it is good practice to eat your breakfast within an hour or so of waking, and it is best not to eat for three or four hours before going to bed. Leave at least two hours between snacks during the day, and four hours between larger meals. Aim to see a sunrise, or watch the sun setting at least once a month – this will help to set your inner timetable – and do some moonbathing whenever there is a full moon. Make time for your own rest, enjoyment and pleasure, and keep some solitary time when you can be alone with yourself. As far as possible stick to a routine; the body finds this comforting and it provides a sense of security that is vital when you are busy or stressed.

Be prepared to experience occasional energy bursts and slumps. Whenever possible, respond to these by stopping what you are doing and taking a five minute break. Choose one of the breathing techniques and spend a minute or two doing it. This may well be enough in itself to balance you. If you have excess energy, use it by doing something physically exerting, or close your eyes and visualise yourself sliding down a long ski slope. Feel how smooth the run is, and enjoy the cooling breeze as it whooshes past you in your rapid descent. Enjoy the pleasure of reaching the bottom of the run where the ground is level and you feel renewed and refreshed. The more intense you make your visualisation, the more real its benefits and after-effects. If you are feeling low, a piece of fruit or a warm drink will often revive your energy. Or you can close your eyes and imagine yourself gathering energy into your body with each fresh breath that you take. Put your hands over your naval to anchor you and help you focus on the reservoir where this energy will be stored.

REWARDS

It is very important that you reward yourself, if possible with a non-food treat, every day. Each day that you do something wonderful for yourself, you can celebrate that in a special way. Be sure to do it.

EATING OUT

Plan ahead and there should be no problems when you eat out. If you are on the Re-Energising Step of your diet and eating every few hours, make sure that the timing works for you; either eat a small meal before you go, and have a small meal when you get there, or plan to eat afterwards. Keep to your routine, and it will only enhance your experience at this time.

Menu choices should not present any difficulties. Most places will provide vegetables or vegetable dishes, and will be happy to make a warm salad and serve your choice of dressing separately. If you are eating animal proteins, you will often find free-range choices marked on the menu, and ask for your food to be grilled, barbecued or roasted.

Asian and Oriental restaurants offer a wide choice of options with a range of vegetable, tofu, rice and noodle dishes. Avoid very hot or creamy curries, and deep fried foods. Latin American choices include beans, corn and crudités with dips, but avoid anything too spicy or cheesy. French/Italian/English restaurants will offer good salad and vegetable choices as well as plain grilled foods and pastas. Again, steer clear of heavy cream sauces. Snack bars often include cooked or roasted vegetable salads and these are good with rice, or as a filling for pitta bread.

During this month of change, choose new restaurants if you possibly can, and order different dishes than you normally would. Endeavour to stick to the step rules and guidelines in the diet as much as possible. Always sit in a non-smoking section.

Finding something to do with your hands is easy if there is bread on the table to crumb, a glass to cradle, or even a napkin that can be knotted on your lap. The challenge here will be to relate and converse with your fellow diners without the usual diversion or camouflage. Treat this as a new event; one that you can enjoy and that will take you a step closer to intimacy. Do not panic, and remember that a little awkwardness is alright in a new situation.

VISITING FRIENDS

When you go to visit friends, let them know ahead of time about your changed circumstances. You may not want to visit a smoker's household while you are following this diet, and until your body and your resolve are feeling strong and clear. Let your hosts know about your diet and what they can do to accommodate you. Often this is as simple as preparing one portion apart from the others, or avoiding one or two ingredients. You can always offer to bring a dish yourself, and if you bring enough to share, it will become part of the meal. One patient of mine offered to cook the meal for her friends – a wonderfully welcome gesture. She prepared a lovely menu from her agreed food list, and did not have to mention that she was following a diet at all.

If you let your friends know about your current plans they will be sure to support and encourage you, but if you do not want to discuss it, it might be best to forewarn them. You do not have to say why you are following a different diet – the choice is yours.

TRAVELLING

Prepare ahead when travelling, and stock up with a good supply of emergency snacks in case your restaurant choices are limited. If you are travelling by train or on shorter distances, plan your timetable so that you can eat before and after your journey, or take a packed lunch with you. Plane journeys often offer quite good meals, and you may be able to enjoy in-flight service without too many changes. It is good advice to keep a snack or two with you when you are going on shorter journeys, or in the car, just in case.

If you are going to be travelling and away from home, stick to your diet and your routine as much as possible. Keep this book with you, and review your food choices at the start of each day to make sure you are clear about your menu choices. If you will have cooking facilities, then take some basic ingredients with you to make sure you have everything to hand. If travelling into other time zones, start your visit with a one-day cleanse – it will help your body adjust itself to the new schedule. Repeat this when you return to home.

SHOPPING

Before you begin each step of the *Just Quit!* diet, read through the directions and check out the lists of foods to choose from. You may find some unusual items such as grains, seaweeds and perhaps some spices or herbs that you do not have in your store cupboard. These can all be found in specialist, health food and Oriental stores.

Health food stores will be a good source for short grain, and wholegrain rice. Basmati rice is also available from Oriental and Asian supermarkets. Wild rice is higher in protein and more warming to the body. It is best used in smaller quantities, or mixed with Basmati. Barley is also widely available, and pot barley is the refined type of pearl barley. It is an excellent source of fibre, calcium and iron, and has a gentle diuretic quality making it a very valuable addition to the diet at this time. Buckwheat is another grain that is very warming and can provide a tasty alternative to rice dishes. This and bulghur wheat, millet and couscous are all warming and make excellent alternatives to widen your diet. Oats are readily available and do wonders for balancing energy swings and calming nerves. They are a rich source of protein as well as minerals and iron. Rye is another suggested grain, and you can find this in crispbreads as well as in grain form. It is excellent when sprouted, or the flour can be substituted for wheat to give a rougher texture.

All sea vegetables or seaweeds contain large amounts of vitamins and minerals. They support thyroid function, being rich in iodine and trace minerals, and so will help support your metabolism. They are usually bought dried, and can be reconstituted by soaking in a little water before using. Choose arame and hijiki to help regulate blood sugar levels, and nori for its protein and delicious taste and texture. Do not soak nori – instead toast the thin sheets over a flame until it becomes crisp. Wakame is a good blood cleanser that needs cooking, and is best added to soups or cooked with grains.

Umeboshi plums are pickled, salted Japanese plums that have a markedly positive effect on digestion. Taken in small amounts they blast the taste buds awake (see page 85). These can be found in Oriental stores and many health food shops.

When you are shopping for fresh fruit and vegetables, remember to include fresh herbs, and other foods like garlic and ginger deserve a permanent place on your shopping list.

Remember that there is no need in your diet right now for additives, flavourings, colourings, synthetic stabilisers, chemical dustings, and any foods that only have a number. If you do not recognise or cannot pronounce an ingredient, leave it.

SPROUTING NUTS AND SEEDS

Step 2 requires you to include a number of different sprouted nuts and seeds. This is easily done at home. Place a selection in a glass jar that you can cover with a clean tea towel or kitchen paper, and rinse with warm water two or three times each day. Keep on a windowsill in the kitchen, and do not let them get too cold. You can buy sprouters which will let you grow two or three layers of sprouts in a container of trays, or you can use more than one jar to keep varieties separate. Most sprouts will be ready to eat within three to five days.

STEP ONE - CLEANSING

This is the first step to cleansing your system. Taking a rest from regular foods and meal customs will help shake loose any old habit patterns that are connected with mealtimes. The fast cleanse will also work to speed toxins from your system and give you a much needed energy boost. It lasts for three days, and the foods chosen will all work to heal various aspects of your body, generally focusing on your mucus membranes, increasing Vitamin C levels and supporting your kidneys and the body's routes of elimination.

Feel free to choose whatever foods you like from those listed – let your taste buds guide you. All the foods have been carefully chosen, but if you have a firm favourite that is not on the list, or feel a real craving for a different fruit, then follow your hunches. Do not be surprised if you find that your likes and dislikes change during this time, so be open minded and consider tasting a few things you might otherwise pass over. Do not be tempted to skip eating altogether unless you are used to fasting. Let the foods do the work of detoxifying your system and returning you to full health and energy.

You must cleanse in order to move on and create space for new and good things to enter your life. This is the ideal way to begin different health habits, but you may also like to return to this healing step at any time. If you are finding it especially beneficial, and it is providing you with all the energy that you need, you can continue the cleansing diet for up to one week. It is most useful if you are feeling in need of a burst of energy, or to manage the transition from one way of eating to another. It is also great when travelling and for relieving pressure during times of stress. One of the great benefits of eating raw food is that it is quite freely available. It is also as nature intended it, and delivers maximum nutrition and energy just when you need it.

Make sure that the foods you select for this cleansing are of the highest possible quality, and are as fresh as possible. Choose naturally or organically grown fruit wherever possible. Make this a gift to yourself that will mark the beginning of choosing top quality nutrition and nurturing in all that you do. Looking after yourself in this way is a real act of grace.

On Day One of your diet you will be eating a wide variety of fresh fruits, and can eat them as often and in whatever quantity you like, provided you do really enjoy them – it is important that you eat because you want or need the energy, not because you want something to do, or are used to putting something in your mouth. Remember to check that you actually want to eat what you choose by closing your eyes for a moment, and imagining the food already in your stomach. See how good it feels, and if it has satisfied your desire. If it has, then go right ahead and eat it. If not, look elsewhere for satisfaction, and come back to the food after 30 minutes.

Day Two sees you simplifying your diet still further as you choose just one fruit, and eat that as often as you like, and when you feel like it, throughout the day. This makes the job of digestion even easier for your body, and means that it can direct its energy towards any immediate healing work that is needed, while being sure to receive adequate nutrients. Listen to your body, and continue to ensure that it is food you want, and not some other satisfaction.

On Day Three you will be able to broaden the variety of foods again, this time choosing from a range of fruits and some vegetables, and adding yoghurt. The job of digestion is made easy by juicing everything you are going to eat. This delivers large amounts of valuable nutrients in a delicious and targeted way. It will also provide you with extra Vitamin C to speed elimination and healing, and give you an additional energy boost.

A juice extractor is a modest but very valuable investment. However, if you do not have one, then many of the fresh juice recipes can be made in a liquidator, pressed, or squeezed. Do not be tempted to rely on bought cartons of commercially produced juice except where indicated.

Throughout the three days you will be drinking large amounts of water to flush out your system. This will give you a feeling of fullness too. Other drinks are included, such as herbal teas that will warm you and aid digestion, and lemon barley water which acts as a mild diuretic. It is important that you drink something, even if it is just a small glass of water, every two hours. If you are feeling the cold, then having a cup of herbal tea or hot water will warm and comfort you. This is invaluable, especially during the colder months. The drinks you choose are as important a part of your nutrition at this time as the foods themselves, so enjoy the experience of being nourished in these different ways.

Balance the cleansing diet by using this time to clear out other areas of your life, so that the energy of change can manifest itself throughout your life. Use the opportunity to tidy your desk, clear out your store cupboards, and tie up any loose ends in your relationships. Cleanse yourself energetically by closing your eyes and seeing a large feather gently sweep any darkness or negativity away from your body and the area surrounding you. Watch it be gently and effectively banished from your vicinity. Then take a moment to feel the change and notice how refreshed and settled you are. Do this whenever you feel the need to be rid of any negativity, and to reinforce the physical work of your body during this detoxification process.

DAY ONE

Today the focus will be on cleansing your system. Eat freely, choosing as many foods as you like from the list below. If you feel like munching your way through the day, that is fine, but if regular meal-breaks suit you better, then leave two hours between these fruit meals. If you do not know which suits you, follow your appetite, and eat when you feel like it. Do not just put a food in your mouth because you want something to do. Close your eyes, imagine it in your stomach, and identify how you feel. Then assess whether you really want the food, or whether you want to do something else instead.

FOODS TO CHOOSE FROM:

grapes
pineapple
mango
papaya
lychees
cherries
apricots
kiwi fruit
apples
pears
ugli fruit

Choose fruits that are ripe and look good, and eat them fresh and uncooked.

The following foods need to be eaten in moderation – add a little for some variety, because they are in season and look good, or if you simply cannot resist:

peaches
all the berries
bananas (maximum of one a day)

DRINKS

cold water – still, not fizzy
Hot Water with Cardamom (see recipe below)
herbal teas: chamomile, peppermint, lemon balm,
Lemon Barley Water (see recipe below)

Have something to drink every two hours, even if you do not feel thirsty – just have a small amount.

RECIPES

HOT WATER WITH CARDAMOM

Boil water and pour into your cup. Add one cardamom pod and leave for five minutes before drinking. This gives a lovely subtle flavour to the water and will warm you and encourage digestion, as well as pleasing your taste buds. Afterwards, you can chew on the pod and swallow the seeds to continue to experience the taste and the benefits. It will also cleanse your breath.

LEMON BARLEY WATER

1 tbsp pearl barley
2 pints water
1 lemon
1/2 tsp honey
2 grains salt

Wash the barley, and add to the water. Place in a saucepan and bring to the boil. Turn off, cover, and leave to stand for 15 minutes. Strain, discarding the barley, and add the juice of the lemon, the honey and the salt. Stir well, and add a little grated or slivered lemon zest.

TIMETABLE NOTES FOR THE DAY

On rising:
Remember to do your chosen breathing exercise
Take your Taste Bud Treat
Have a drink
Make sure you eat breakfast

Throughout the day:
Drink at least every two hours
Leave two hours between meal times
Do not eat after 7.30pm
Walk for five minutes

Undertake one symbolic act, such as clearing out a drawer, raking up some leaves, sorting your wardrobe, or bringing order to an area of clutter, and reinforce the energy of cleansing in your life.

DAY TWO

Today you will be reinforcing the work you began yesterday, and focusing on specific cleansing of your system. Choose one fruit from the list below, and eat as much of that as you like throughout today. Choose a fruit that you really like, and make sure that you can have lots of it. The key to this day is sticking to the one fruit, so the season and your local supermarket may dictate what is available to you. Wherever possible pick fruits that have been naturally or organically grown. Do not try to stick to regular mealtimes, eat when you feel hungry, and when you feel like it. Continue to drink something every two hours.

FOODS

red or black grapes – a good choice if you tend to like to pick at food, or experience energy slumps

pineapple – very good for meat eaters, but less good if you are very overweight

mango – this is a delicious, if expensive, choice – make sure the fruit is ripe

cherries – very good for dealing with any arthritic concerns

apples – excellent cleansers that work to soothe the gut

pears – very good cleansers with a good mineral balance

melon – watermelon, ogens or charantais – high energy cleansers that will soothe an irritated bowel

apricots – sweet and gentle on the stomach, a rich source of Vitamin A

kiwi fruit – easy to eat and high in Vitamin C

DRINKS

water (hot or cold)

herbal teas: chamomile, fennel
Fenugreek Tea (see recipe below)
Hot Ginger Tea (see recipe below)

Have something to drink every two hours, even if you are not thirsty. Take a hot drink each time you eat if you have chosen apples, pears or any of the three melons for your fruit fast.

RECIPES

FENUGREEK TEA

1 tsp fenugreek seeds
2 cups water
1/4 tsp blackstrap molasses

Add the seeds to the water in a saucepan and bring to the boil. Cook for two minutes, then turn off the heat and leave to stand, covered, for five minutes. Strain, discarding the seeds, and stir in the molasses, making sure it is quite dissolved. This is an excellent tonic and will pep up any flagging energy levels.

HOT GINGER TEA

1 pint water
1 inch fresh ginger root
1 slice of lemon
1/4 tsp honey

Bring the water to the boil in a saucepan, and slice the ginger root. When the water is boiling, add the sliced ginger, cover, and reduce the heat to a simmer. Cook for 20 minutes then strain, discarding the ginger. Stir in the honey and add the slice of lemon. This is excellent on cold, wet days, and will strengthen your digestion.

TIMETABLE NOTES FOR THE DAY

On rising:
Remember to do your chosen breathing exercise
Take your Taste Bud Treat
Have a drink

Throughout the day:
Drink at least every two hours
Eat whenever you feel hungry
Do not eat after 9.00pm
Walk for five minutes
Make a list of physical activities that you will undertake within the next week, and schedule time for them in your diary.

DAY THREE

Today your focus will be on resting your digestion, making sure you have all the energy you need, and continuing the work of detoxifying your system. This is the last day of Step 1, and is crucial in order to make the transition to the next step of the diet an easy one. It is also a particularly tasty day, and one that you can choose to repeat if you find it suits you. This is one of the easiest and most adaptable days so you can return to it for an energy boost, or to give your system a rest, whenever you choose.

Choose any or all of the foods listed, and juice them. Juicing is an easy way to obtain maximum benefit from fruits and vegetables. It will provide you with extra Vitamin C to speed elimination and healing, and give you an energy boost. Make sure you have a juice blend, or a neutral drink from the list below, every two hours. Take the juices with added water, diluting them half and half, to make it easier on your stomach. Make sure that you 'chew' the juice – holding it in your mouth for a moment to enable the important first stage of digestion. Drink all fresh juices as soon as possible after preparation. You begin to lose vitamins and enzymes after as little as one minute!

FOODS

Choose any of the foods below, but only have them juiced, do not eat them whole.

apples
pears
pineapple **
grapefruit **
grapes
apricots
kiwi fruit
berries (in small amounts only)
carrot
fennel
celery
lettuce
parsley
beetroot **
watercress

** These juices can be bought in cartons or bottles, otherwise, juice your own.

For your last juice blend of the day you can stir in some natural live goat's or sheep's yoghurt if you choose. Pick an organic brand if you can. Beat it in to the prepared juice to add thickness and flavour, as a digestive aid, and to help prepare you for sleep. This will also prepare your digestion for the return to solid food tomorrow.

DRINKS

In addition to the individual juices and juice blends, choose:

water (hot or cold)
Coriander and Ginger Tonic (see page 102)
Moroccan Mint Tea (see page 103)

RECIPES

Most fruits can be juiced and taste wonderful on their own. Good combinations include:
- *apple, pear and carrot*
- *carrot, apple and celery*
- *pineapple and grapefruit*
- *fennel, celery and watercress*
- *pineapple, apple and pear*
- *grape, carrot and parsley*

Remember to dilute all juices with an equal amount of still water.

Add a small piece of beetroot, or a splash of beetroot juice to any of the juices to stimulate your liver and add a pleasing earthiness to the taste. This also does wonders for the colour.

Add a small slice of pineapple to any of the fruit juices to sweeten and encourage digestion.

Pineapple and grapefruit juice is a wonderful cleanser that will encourage your liver and gall bladder, and tastes fantastic.

Apple, lettuce and grapes make for a gentle and easy breakfast juice.

Fennel, carrot and pear combine well with yoghurt for your final juice of the day.

Combine pineapple and apricots with water in a blender, and top with a few ripe berries for a light, sweet juice that is packed with energy.

CORIANDER AND GINGER TONIC

1 tbsp coriander seeds
1/2 piece of fresh ginger root

1 pint water
1/2 lemon
1/4 tsp honey

Add the coriander seed to a saucepan with the water and bring to the boil. Add the finely chopped or grated ginger, cover, and simmer for 10 minutes. Remove from the heat, and add the sliced lemon. Leave to stand for about three minutes, then stir in the honey making sure it is well dissolved. This is a warming and healing drink that is perfect and tasty way to banish any early cold-type symptoms.

MOROCCAN MINT TEA

1 cup of fresh mint leaves or 2 peppermint tea bags
1 pint water
1/2 tsp cinnamon
1/4 tsp honey
pinch of dried ginger

Cram the fresh mint leaves into a pot and cover with the boiled water, or use the tea bags. Steep for 3-10 minutes, depending on how strong you like the flavour to be. Mint loses its fresh, cool edge after about three minutes, but the resultant taste is still to many people's liking. Strain, discarding the mint, and stir in the cinnamon and honey, and add the pinch of dried ginger just before drinking. A lovely twist on a traditional drink that will treat your taste buds.

TIMETABLE NOTES FOR EACH DAY

On rising:
Keep to your early morning routine of breathing exercises, etc.,
Have a Taste Bud Treat
Have a breakfast juice

Throughout the day:
Drink a juice or have a glass of water or other neutral drink from the list provided every two hours

Do not have anything after 9.00pm
Enjoy a little exercise

CONGRATULATIONS. You have completed Step 1 of the *Just Quit!* diet. Make sure you reward yourself with a non-food treat or celebration of some kind. Continue your good work and move directly on to Step 2. It is full of tasty treats and snacks and opens up a new variety of foods and ways of eating that will take you further towards restoring balance and harmony to your system.

STEP TWO -
RE-ENERGISING

After the quick blast of Vitamin C and cleansing from Step 1, Step 2 will provide you with a sustained and regular intake of foods to soothe jangled nerves and equip your body to manage the stress of changed habit patterns. This step is all about re-energising your system and balancing out blood sugar levels. It will address mineral deficiencies and provide you with maximum amounts of calcium and B-vitamins to settle your nerves. To achieve all of this, you will be focusing on eating something from the recommended food lists every 2 1/2 – 3 hours. A combination of healthy and tasty snacks, and meals that are smaller than you are used to eating, will ensure that you provide your body with good nutrition as regularly as possible. The food choices are also high in Vitamin E, which amongst a host of other good deeds for your body will combat skin dryness (great for the face after contact with all that smoke), and meet any residual EFA (Essential Fatty Acid) deficiency.

The food lists contain a wide choice, with the main focus on grains, nuts and seeds to ensure maximum B-vitamins and mineral levels, and also the sustained energy that grains provide. Much attention is also paid to the taste and flavour of meals so that you are getting the greatest satisfaction at this first important stage of digestion. Fire is included in the intensity of barbecued, chargrilled and roasted foods, which give a real intensity of smoky flavour. Most of the meals are warming and will stimulate your digestion and provide lots of energy. When adequate amounts of grains are eaten, the levels of tryptophan in the brain rise. This is responsible for the production of serotonin and will generate feelings of calm and well-being.

Remember that you need to eat breakfast every day. This is one of the most valuable things you can do for your body. It will provide you with the energy you need to make a good start to the day and will ensure that you are not left looking for a quick-fix or a pick-me-up just an hour or two into the day.

Keep drinking something every two hours. It does not have to be in any great quantity, just choose a glass of water, or any of the drinks from the food lists on the next pages.

Do not go for more than three hours without eating something. Eating every 2 1/2 – 3 hours means your daily timetable will look something like this:

> breakfast 7.30am
> snack 10.00am
> lunch 12.30pm
> snack 3.00pm
> dinner 6.00pm
> snack 8.30pm

Adjust this if you get up earlier or later, but do not snack on anything after 10pm, and make sure you have two hours to digest your food before going to bed. This can be followed quite easily if you plan an early lunch and can have an early dinner too. If not, stick as closely as possible to the time interval, perhaps having a more substantial snack at mid-afternoon and a light snack at 6.00pm, and some more substantial food at 8.30pm. Never go past these eating times – have some form of snack if you cannot have a small meal. This may seem odd at first, but is a valuable step in helping your body trust that you will provide it with regular, good nutrition.

It is very important that you keep your energy levels constant, and that your body learns to receive its energy from the foods you are eating. The safeguards here are that you measure the quantity of snacks that you take, and never keep more than one small bowl of something near you – this is not a recipe for becoming a couch potato! You should never have more than three snacks in a day, and never abuse your system by eating more often than every two hours.

As before, make sure that you want the food before each snack by taking a deep breath, closing your eyes, and imagining the food already in your stomach. See how it feels, and whether you really want it. If you do, go right ahead, but if not, then find some other way to satisfy your self. If your appetite is not good, have very small snacks, but do still continue to have them.

You will be following this step of the diet for between 7-10 days. If you are happy with it, you can extend it up to two weeks, but there is more work to be done, and Step 3 has a valuable role to play in stabilising your health. Women should come back to this step for three days prior to each period to relieve any residual pre-menstrual symptoms.

You will find small amounts of oil or ghee used in some of the recipes and you can eat up to one tablespoon a day of good quality, cold-pressed oil, or ghee. Choose olive, safflower or sunflower oils unless you have your own favourite. You can buy ghee in most Asian stores and many supermarkets, or make your own very easily using 1 lb of unsalted butter.

MAKING GHEE

Place this in a heavy non-aluminium saucepan that is not non-stick, and heat on the lowest setting for more than five minutes, or until the butter has separated, is gently bubbling, and the solids in the bottom are just beginning to turn slightly deeper in colour. Strain through a metal sieve covered with muslin, leaving the solids behind. This will keep for three months in the fridge, or for up to three weeks without.

Salt is kept to a minimum and must not be left on the table for you to add to cooked meals! Small amounts appear in some of the recipes and you can add up to half a teaspoon each day to cooking, not for sprinkling on later. Sea vegetables add a great flavour to meals, and with the recommendations given for flavours, herbs and spices you should not miss salt much at all.

Sugar is also kept to a minimum. A few grains of muscovado or raw cane sugar is added occasionally in cooking, but you will need to limit yourself to one teaspoon each day.

The food and menu suggestions do not include any animal-based meals. You can barbecue, roast or grill foods that you usually eat if you notice any cravings or feel the lack of them. Add these to the recommended foods, and include them not more than once a day.

DAYS FOUR – FOURTEEN

Today, and for the next 7-10 days, your work will be to provide your body with good sources of physical energy every 2 1/2 – 3 hours. The foods you choose will be high in the necessary fibre, vitamins and minerals to soothe your system and ease your nerves. You can eat your own favourite dishes if they stick to the food list ingredients, but make your meals a little smaller than you would usually, bearing in mind that you will be eating again within three hours.

• Make sure that you have breakfast every day within one hour of getting up, and do not go for more than three hours without eating something from the following food lists.
• Continue having something to drink every two hours.
• Do not have more than three snacks in any day, and always make sure you leave two hours between eating.
• Make sure each meal you have features a grain, and ensure cooking methods are as tasty as possible – choose barbecued, chargrilled and roasted foods for maximum flavour.
• Eat five portions of fruit or vegetables every day and include green, leafy vegetables at least once a day.
• Eat sprouts at least once a day.
• Eat a sea vegetable every day.
• Chew everything very well.

FOODS TO CHOOSE FROM

Vegetables: asparagus, aubergines, avocados, beetroot, broccoli, cabbage – red, white, savoy, winter – carrots, chard, celery, chicory, endive, courgette, fennel, garlic, kale, lettuce, leeks, marrow, mustard and cress, onions, parsnips, peas – and sugar snap and mange tout – potatoes, spring greens, spinach, squash – butternut, patty pans, etc. – swedes, turnips, watercress, hijiki, arame, dulse, nori, and any other seaweeds or sea vegetables

Fruits: apples, apricots, bananas (not more than one a day), berries (sweet, not sour such as redcurrants, and only once a day), cherries, dates, dried fruits, figs, grapes, grapefruit, ugli fruit, melons – watermelon, charantais and ogen – kiwi fruit, lychee, mango, papaya, passion fruit, pomegranate, lime and lemon (not more than once a day)

Sprouts: aduki, alfalfa, chickpeas, buckwheat, fenugreek, mung beans, peas, radish, rye, sunflower seeds

Flowers: nasturtiums, marigolds, cowslips

Grains: barley, couscous, buckwheat, bulghur wheat, millet, oats, rice – wholegrain, short grain brown rice, basmati, wild – rice noodles, rye. Eat wheat in moderation – not more than once every other day, and avoid yeast. This means no regular bread, but pitta, naan, soda, etc. Include oat cakes, rice cakes, crispbreads, crackers, bagels and popadoms, but read the labels to be sure – even some rye breads contain wheat

Beans: aduki beans, chickpeas, mung beans, red lentils

Nuts and Seeds: caraway, poppy, pumpkin, sesame, sunflower, almond, brazil nuts, walnuts, pecans, pine nuts, unsalted pistachios

Herbs and Spices: basil, bay, dill, oregano, parsley, mint, rosemary, sage, thyme, cinnamon, coriander, cumin, mustard seeds, saffron, turmeric, pepper

Dairy: goat's and sheep's milk, live yoghurt and cheese in small amounts (not more than once every other day), rice, oat, soya and other grain milks daily. If you eat eggs, you can have two a week.

DRINKS

Water (hot and cold) – still, not fizzy
Dilute fresh fruit and vegetable juices
Rosehip Tea (High in Vitamin C and a treat in its strong, cheery red colour)
Rosehip and Hibiscus
Red Zinger herbal tea blend
Any drinks from Step 1
Hot Apple Cider (see page 130)
Night-Time Soothers (see page 130)

RECIPES

BREAKFASTS

A warming breakfast is a good idea, especially during the cold weather, but if you cannot manage that then have a hot drink from your list before you eat. Consider adding warmed milk to your corn-flakes to make a hot meal.

DRIED FRUIT COMPOTE

Choose from a selection of dried fruits that do not contain sulpher. Organic choices are more healthful, but if these are not available then rinse the dried fruits well in warm water before soaking.

Dried apples, pears, peaches, apricots, mango and figs make a stunning combination. Take a small bowl of the mixed fruits and soak in three times the amount of water in a lidded saucepan overnight. In the morning, heat the fruit through in the remaining liquid (you will see that much of it has been absorbed, and the fruit will be soft, plumped up and delicious). Serve with a scattering of sesame seeds on top and a spoonful of live yoghurt.

STEWED FRUIT

1 large cooking apple
1/2 tsp cinnamon
3 tbsp water
1/4 tsp honey or muscovado sugar

Peel, core and slice the apple. Add to a saucepan with the water and cinnamon, and cover and cook over a low heat for 10-15 minutes. Remove from the heat and stir in the honey or sugar. Serve straight away, or leave to cool.

Apricots are delicious cooked in this way. Add a little lemon juice, and substitute two cloves for the cinnamon.

FRESH FRUIT SAUCE

Berries and other soft fruits make a lovely, colourful sauce that can be eaten on its own or poured over rice and other grains.

Put two cups of fruit in a saucepan with 1/4 cup of water and cook very gently for about 10 minutes. Liquidate to smooth out still further, and add honey. Add 1/8 cup of yoghurt to make a delicious smoothie.

SPICY PORRIDGE

1 cup oat flakes
2 1/2 cups of water (or follow directions on packet)
1/4 tsp salt
1/4 tsp ground cinnamon
1/8 tsp powdered ginger
1/4 cup any milk except cow's
1/4 tsp honey or cane sugar

Add the oat flakes and salt to the water and cook as directed, or bring to the boil, then turn down to a simmer and stir frequently for 3-10 minutes or until the oats are soft and well cooked. Stir in the cinnamon and ginger, then remove from the heat and cover and leave for 1-2 minutes to let the flavours blend. Stir in the milk and honey or sugar, and enjoy.

This warming breakfast dish is wonderfully warming on a cold winter day, and makes a good snack or light supper dish too.

BREAKFAST RICE

This is an excellent way of eating up last night's cooked rice.

1 cup of cooked rice
1 cup of any milk except cow's
1/4 cup raisins
1/4 cup walnuts or blanched almonds
1/2 tsp ground cinnamon

Put the rice and milk in a saucepan with the raisins and warm gently. Cook for 4-5 minutes, then add the nuts and the cinnamon. Stir in well, then leave to warm through for another minute before serving.

SPICY TOFU

This is a great alternative to scrambled eggs, and one that will delight your taste buds. Even those people who do not like tofu seem to like it when it is cooked this way.

8 oz block of tofu
1 tbsp olive or sunflower oil or ghee
1 garlic clove, crushed
1/8 inch piece of fresh ginger root peeled and grated
1/4 tsp powdered turmeric
1/4 tsp grain mustard
1/4 tsp sea salt
1/4 tsp black pepper
1/8 tsp ground cumin

Heat the oil or ghee in a pan, and add the crushed garlic clove. Cook for a moment, without letting it colour, and then add the tofu, mashing it in the pan until it is in small pieces. Add the rest of the ingredients, stirring well to make sure they are mixed, and cook for 3-5 minutes.

This is a delicious way to spice up the delicate flavour of tofu. Serve it for breakfast on some warmed pitta bread, or with rice as a light lunch.

SNACKS

bunch of sweet black or red grapes
bowl of lychees
handful of cherries
3 apricots
banana (not more than one a day)

peach
mango
papaya
2 pineapple slices
1 apple
few berries – strawberry, raspberry, blueberry
2 kiwi fruit
red grapefruit
pomegranate
3 figs
slice of melon (with watermelon, add a pinch of black pepper to help digestion)
6 dates
brazil nuts, walnuts
pistachio nuts
3 cardamom seeds in their shells
5 rice cakes
2 oat cakes
deep fried seaweed

Try the following from the recipe selection:
Digestive Mix
Dry Roasted Peanuts
Spiced Sunflower Seeds
Roasted Pumpkin Seeds
Trail Mix
Dried Apricots and Brazil Nuts
Hydrated Raisins
Soaked Almonds
Almond Stuffed Dates
Honey and Sesame Treats

DIGESTIVE MIX

1 tbsp fennel seeds
1 tbsp cumin seeds
1 tbsp coriander seeds

small pinch of salt
small pinch of muscovado or raw cane sugar

Heat a heavy-bottomed pan, and add the seeds. Cook for about one minute – just long enough for the seeds to release their aroma and begin to brown. Immediately turn into a cool bowl and add a pinch of salt and a pinch of sugar. Mix together and allow to cool.

This is an excellent snack for the end of the day, or it can also be taken after a meal to aid digestion.

DRY ROASTED PEANUTS

1 cup of peanuts
1/2 tsp garlic powder
1/2 tsp chilli powder
1/2 tsp ground coriander

Heat a heavy bottomed pan, and add the peanuts. Cook for about one minute – just long enough for the peanuts to begin to brown, then add the garlic, chilli and coriander powders. Turn off the heat, and mix in the pan. Leave to cool, then turn into a serving bowl.

SPICED SUNFLOWER SEEDS

1 cup of sunflower seeds
1/2 tsp curry powder or garam masala
3-5 grains fenugreek
1/2 tsp ground coriander

Heat a heavy-bottomed pan and add the fenugreek grains. Cook for about 30 seconds – until the flavour is released. Add the sunflower seeds and cook for a further 3-5 minutes, until browned and starting to pop. Sprinkle on the curry powder or garam masala and coriander, and turn into a serving bowl.

This also makes a great topping for breakfast porridge.

ROASTED PUMPKIN SEEDS

1 cup pumpkin seeds
1/2 tsp ground cumin
1 tsp ground coriander
1/4 tsp turmeric

1 tsp soy sauce (Note – this is not on your food lists, but the small amount makes all the difference to this recipe, and should not adversely effect your outcome.)

Heat a heavy-bottomed pan and add all the ingredients except the soy sauce. Mix well and cook for about 5-8 minutes, until the seeds are roasted and brown, and beginning to pop. Sprinkle with soy sauce and turn into a serving bowl.

Add to warm salad for extra texture and minerals, and a delicious flavour.

TRAIL MIX

1/2 cup dried apricots
1/2 cup raisins
3 figs, chopped
3 dates, chopped
1 tbsp sesame seeds
1 tbsp sunflower seeds
1 tbsp pumpkin seeds
1/2 cup almonds
4 brazil nuts, chopped

Prepare the ingredients and mix well together. Add other dried fruits such as apple and pear when in season, or substitute dried mango and papaya for the apricots for a more tropical blend.

DRIED APRICOTS AND BRAZIL NUTS

1 cup dried apricots
1 cup whole brazil nuts, shelled
1 cup hot water

Soak the apricots in the hot water for five minutes, until they just begin to swell. Cool, and then open each apricot carefully, and fill with a brazil nut, rolling it closed again around it.

HYDRATED RAISINS

1 cup raisins
1 cup hot water

Soak raisins in one cup of boiling water for 10 minutes before eating.

SOAKED ALMONDS

6-8 almonds
1 cup hot water

Soak almonds in boiling water for 10 minutes, then handle carefully and remove the skin. This is hard to digest and is best left. Alternatively, soak in cold water overnight, for an early morning snack. Make a calcium rich almond milk by liquidating the nuts together with the liquid after it has been soaked.

ALMOND STUFFED DATES

1 cup dates
1/2 cup of almond slivers

Chop one quarter of the dates very finely, and mix with the almond slivers. This should form a type of paste. Take the remaining dates and carefully open. Stuff the date and almond paste into the cavity and roll closed. Vary this by adding a few soaked raisins or some sesame seeds.

HONEY AND SESAME TREATS

1 cup sesame seeds
1/4 cup tahini or sesame seed paste
1 tsp thick set honey

Mix together the tahini and honey. Use a warmed spoon or knife because this will be very thick and hard to move. Take small teaspoon sized pieces and roll into balls. Roll the balls in fresh or toasted sesame seeds. Leave to set for about 10-15 minutes before eating. If you want to keep these, they will need to be refrigerated.

LIGHT MEALS

ADUKI BEAN SOUP

4 oz aduki beans, soaked in water for three hours or overnight
1 tsp olive or other good oil
1 onion
2 celery stalks
1 carrot
1 clove garlic
1 stick kombu seaweed
1 bay leaf
1 tsp each chopped or dried oregano, thyme and parsley
1 1/2 pints stock or water
salt and pepper

Chop the onion, celery and carrot, and crush the garlic. Heat the oil in a large pan and add the onion and celery, cooking gently for 2-3 minutes. Add the remaining ingredients, except the salt and pepper. Bring to the boil and then simmer with a lid on for one hour. Remove from the heat and add freshly ground pepper and up to half a teaspoon of salt to taste. Cover for 3-5 minutes and let stand before serving to let the flavours develop.

QUICK RED LENTIL SOUP

4 oz red lentils
1 onion
1 carrot
a handful of spinach leaves or other greens, or few bitter salad leaves
pinch of salt and freshly ground black pepper

Place the lentils in a saucepan with the chopped onion and carrot, and the rinsed spinach or greens. (If using salad leaves, add at the end of the cooking time.) Cover with about two pints of water, and bring to the boil. Skim any scum off the surface, then cover and simmer for about 20 minutes, or until the lentils have become soft and mushy, and the carrot is soft. If adding bitter leaves, add them now. Serve with cooked grains, or with mixed grain bread.

MIXED VEGETABLE SOUP

2 tbsp olive or sunflower oil
1 tsp cumin seeds
1 onion
3 sticks of celery
1 carrot
1 summer squash or piece of pumpkin
1 courgette
2-3 new potatoes
2 oz mange tout or sugar snap peas
1 stick kombu seaweed
1 tsp ground cumin
1/4 tsp salt
1/4 tsp ground black pepper

Heat the oil in a pan and when warm add the cumin seeds. Chop the onion and the celery, and add to the pan once the seeds have browned. Cook gently for 3-4 minutes, then add two pints of water and bring to the boil. Chop the carrot, squash and courgette into pieces and quarter the potatoes and add to the pan with the mange-tout or sugar snap peas and the rinsed kombu. Cover and reduce to a simmer, cooking for about 30 minutes. Just before serving stir in the ground cumin, salt and pepper.

Variations:

• Stir in some barley with the celery and onion, and double the amount of water. Cook for one hour, for a tasty thick broth.

• Add a 4 oz piece of tofu to the vegetables half way through the cooking time for extra protein.

GOLDEN SOUP

The rich warming colour of this soup is nourishing in itself!

1 large onion
2 tbsp olive or sunflower oil
3 sticks of celery
2 carrots
1 summer squash or large slice of pumpkin
4 oz sweet corn
piece of wakame seaweed

Slice the pumpkin and remove the seeds. Bake in a hot oven for about 20 minutes, then chop, removing the skin if it is thick. Meanwhile, chop the onion finely, and fry in the oil until just starting to become soft. Add the chopped celery, and continue to cook for a further minute or two. Chop the carrots and squash or pumpkin and add to the pan, coating in the mixture. Cook for one minute, then add about two pints of water. Bring to the boil, then cover, add the rinsed wakame and simmer for 15 minutes. Add the sweet corn and cook for a further 15 minutes. (If using frozen or canned corn, leave it for another 15 minutes before adding.) Cook for a further five minutes, then liquidate.

Serve with a sprinkling of toasted sunflower seeds, or over a small baked onion – sounds odd, but the sweetness adds a deliciousness.

PESTO WITH TOFU

1/2 lb tofu
2 large handfuls fresh basil leaves
1 tbsp olive oil
1 clove garlic, crushed
1 tbsp tahini
3 tbsp water

Steam the tofu for five minutes, then cut into chunks and put in a liquidator. Blitz briefly to break down the pieces, then add all the rest of the ingredients. Do not over-blend or the basil will loose its delicate freshness.

Serve this delicious dip as a topping, or a dip for vegetables.

GRILLED AUBERGINE

1 medium sized aubergine
1 tbsp olive or sunflower oil
1 tbsp olive paté
2 oz fetta or goat's cheese
fresh coriander leaves

Wash the aubergine and slice it very thinly. Brush one side of each slice with a small amount of the oil, or use a spray. Place under a hot grill, oiled side up, and cook until brown. Watch the slices carefully as they can burn very quickly, especially if they are very thin. Take them out and turn each slice over. Top with a little paté and a sliver of cheese. Place back under the grill until the cheese melts and browns. Tear some coriander leaves roughly and settle on top of each slice.

This makes a delicious snack, and can form the basis of a meal if you slice the aubergine length ways. Serve with mixed grains and a warmed salad.

OVEN ROASTED VEGETABLES

1 courgette
1 red onion
3-4 patty pans or 1 small squash
1 medium potato
1 fennel bulb
1 tbsp olive or other oil,
sprigs of thyme and rosemary
black pepper
1/4 tsp nori flakes

Slice all the vegetables into the same size chunks. Heat the oil in an oven proof dish, and toss the vegetables in the warmed oil. Add the herbs, then roast in a medium oven for 30-40 minutes, until the vegetables are brown and have developed a crispy oatside coating. Turn once about midway through the cooking time. Remove from the oven and sprinkle with freshly ground black pepper and the nori flakes.

ROASTED GARLIC

1 head of garlic
1 tbsp olive oil
1 large sprig fresh rosemary or small bunch of thyme

Heat the oven, and put the olive oil in an oven proof dish. Cut the head of garlic in half across its middle. Lay the herbs in the dish and place the garlic on top, cut side down. Roast for about 30 minutes in a moderate oven.

This deliciously pungent and healing dish is a tasty addition to grains and vegetables. Serve one half per person. You can also have this as a snack by squeezing the garlic out and spreading it on to a crispbread or half a toasted bagel, or add it to soup.

BAKED ONION TRAY

5 onions or 2-3 large Spanish onions

1 tbsp olive oil
1 tsp cumin seeds

Peel the onions and cut them in half, then slice them length ways to make crescent shapes. Place in an oven proof dish and pour in the oil. Mix well, then sprinkle the cumin seeds on top. Cook in a hot oven for 15 minutes, then mix well and return to the oven for a further 15-25 minutes or until the onions are sweet and soft and delicious.

Serve with rice or other grains and steamed vegetables topped with a french or herb dressing. This will add a little zip to any plain meals, and is especially good with grains.

ROASTED PARSNIPS

2 large parsnips
1 pint water
1 tbsp olive or other good oil
1 tsp apple juice concentrate

Slice the parsnips into one inch pieces and boil or steam for 3-5 minutes until just starting to become tender. Meanwhile, heat the oil in an ovenproof dish in a moderately hot oven. Drain the parsnips and dry them, then add to the oil, mixing well, and pour on the apple juice concentrate. Roast in the oven for about 30 minutes until sweet and golden.

BAKED SPICY SQUASH

1 butternut squash
1 tsp olive oil
1 clove garlic, crushed
1/4 tsp ground cumin, cinnamon and ginger
black pepper

Cut the squash in half and take out the seeds. Then slice and score the surface of each piece with a knife to make a criss-cross pattern that just breaks the surface. Mix together the garlic, cumin, cinnamon and ginger to make a paste, and rub into the squash slices. Put in an oven proof dish and bake in a hot oven for about 20 minutes, depending on the thickness of the slices, until soft, sweet, spicy and golden in colour. Alternatively, cut quite thin slices and grill or barbecue.

STIR FRY VEGETABLES

1 tbsp olive or other oil
handful of fresh sage leaves
1 large onion
2 carrots
2 celery sticks
1 courgette
1 leek
1/2 inch fresh ginger root
2 cloves garlic
1/4 tsp mustard seeds
1/4 tsp cumin seeds
small handful of nuts or seeds
large handful of mixed sprouts
1 sheet nori, flaked
salt and pepper

Slice the onion, and cut the carrot into thin strips. Slice the celery and courgette and shred the leek. Slice the ginger and garlic very thinly. Heat the oil in a wok or a large, heavy bottomed pan, and drop the sage leaves in. Scoop them out straight away and leave to cool. Add the mustard and cumin seeds, ginger and garlic, letting them flavour the oil while they cook. Do not let them burn. Add the rest of the vegetables except for the sprouts, and cook, turning frequently, for about three minutes. Stir in the sprouts and nuts, and add freshly ground black pepper and a pinch of salt, and sprinkle the toasted and flaked nori on top with the sage leaves which should be crispy and delicious.

GRILLED VEGETABLES

1 courgette
1 leek
1 potato
1 aubergine
1 small celeriac
1 parsnip
1 tbsp olive or other oil
bunches of fresh sage
1 tsp dried oregano
black pepper
1 bunch fresh parsley

Slice the courgette, leek, aubergine and parsnip length ways. Slice the potato and celeriac into thinner slices. Put in a dish and mix thoroughly with the oil, oregano and pepper. Place the sage leaves on the grill, or in a grill-proof dish and lay the vegetables on top. Cook under a high heat, turning once, until the vegetables are brown and crispy. (Watch the aubergines as they can cook very quickly.) Remove from the heat. Chop the parsley up very finely and cover the vegetables with it.

HUMMOUS

4 oz chick peas soaked overnight in three times their quantity of water
1/2 tsp salt
2 tbsp tahini (sesame seed paste)
2-4 garlic cloves, crushed
juice of 1/2 lemon
1 tbsp olive oil
bunch each of mint and coriander chopped.

Drain the chick peas, and place in a saucepan covered in fresh water. Bring to the boil, then simmer gently for about two hours until soft. Turn off the heat and add half a teaspoon of salt, then cover and leave to stand for 10 minutes. Drain, reserving four fluid ounces of the liquid, and put this in a liquidator with the chick peas, salt, tahini, garlic lemon juice and olive oil. Blend and then add some ground black pepper and the fresh herbs.

This is a very moreish snack that is great as a dip with raw vegetables, and makes a wonderful filling for pitta bread.

GREEN BEAN SALAD

8 oz runner beans or chopped french green beans
1 tbsp olive or sunflower oil
1 tbsp mustard
1 tbsp honey
pinch of salt

Cook the beans very well, and while they are cooking mix together the oil, mustard and honey. Drain the beans, and pour the dressing over straight away. Sprinkle a pinch of salt over.

This is delicious with rice or other grains, and will spice up an otherwise dullish meal.

SOSMIX SNACKS

These are so much more tasty and moreish than regular animal sausages. They can be snacked on or used to form a main meal.

1 packet of Sosmix or other seasoned soya mix
1 tbsp milk
2 oz fresh breadcrumbs
oil for frying
1 tbsp Dijon or other mild mustard

Make up the sausages as directed on the packet, using slightly less water than suggested. When rehydrated form into small balls. Put the milk in a saucer, and the breadcrumbs in another. Pass the sosmix balls through the milk, and cover in the breadcrumbs, then fry until brown and crispy. Serve with a large dab of mustard.

GRAINS

BASIC RICE

4 oz basmati rice
1/2 tsp salt
1/2 tsp turmeric
1 pint water

Wash the rice very well and place in a saucepan of boiling water with the salt. Bring to the boil and skim off the starch. Add the turmeric. Cover and simmer for 10-15 minutes, then strain.

BASMATI RICE

1 tsp olive or sunflower oil
1/2 tsp cumin seeds
1/2 tsp black mustard seeds
4 oz basmati or other white rice
1/2 tsp sea salt
1/2 tsp black pepper

Heat the oil in a pan, and add the cumin seeds and the black mustard seeds. Wash the rice very well, and add to the pan once the mustard seeds start to pop and the cumin has turned brown. Add the salt and about one pint of water. Bring to the boil, then cover and simmer for 10 minutes. Fork through and add the black pepper just before serving.

BROWN RICE

4 oz brown short grain rice
2 pints water

Rinse the rice very well. Place in a pan with the cold water and bring to the boil. Skim the surface, and cover and simmer over a low heat for about 40 minutes or until cooked. Try not to stir during cooking. Once done, rinse with boiling water and serve.

Variation: Cook equal amounts of brown rice and barley together

BROWN RICE AND BARLEY

4 oz brown short grain rice
4 oz pearl barley
2 pints water

Mix the grains together and rinse well. Follow directions for Brown Rice.

Variation: substitute wild rice for the barley to add protein and texture.

TASTY COUSCOUS WITH VEGETABLES

8 oz couscous
1 pint stock
4 oz cooked chick peas
1 oz nori, flaked
2 oz dried apricots
1 oz flaked almonds
1 large bunch fresh mint leaves, and one of coriander

Place the couscous in a large bowl and pour the warmed stock over it. Leave to stand for about 10 minutes, and the liquid will be absorbed. Mix in the chick peas and the apricots. Chop the fresh herbs finely, and mix in with the flaked nori and almonds.

NUTTY TABBOULEH

5 oz cracked bulghur wheat
bunch of spring onions
3 cloves of garlic, chopped or crushed
3 tbsp fresh mint
3 tbsp fresh coriander
1 tbsp fresh lemon balm
1 small courgette
1/2 cup pine nuts, toasted

1/2 cup blanched almonds, slivered and toasted
1/4 cup walnuts, broken in pieces
juice of 1 lemon
1 tbsp olive oil

Soak the wheat in a bowl of cold water for an hour, then drain and leave to dry. Chop the spring onions finely with the courgette and herbs. Mix together with the dried bulghur wheat and dress with the olive oil and lemon juice. Leave to stand for an hour to let the flavours deepen, then mix in the nuts.

COOKED TABBOULEH

5 oz cracked bulghur wheat
1 onion
3 cloves garlic, chopped or crushed
1 leek
1 carrot
1 tablespoon olive oil
1 bunch asparagus
1 large bunch fresh parsley
water

Cook the wheat by covering with boiling water and heating in a saucepan for 10-15 minutes. Drain and keep warm to mix in with the vegetables when they are cooked. Roughly chop the onion and heat with the garlic in a pan until transluscent and soft. Add the shredded leek and finely chopped carrot and two tablespoons of water. Cook for a further five minutes, then add the asparagus broken or cut into one inch pieces. Cover and cook until these are soft. Chop the parsley, then mix all the ingredients together while they are still warm.

BEVERAGES

HOT APPLE CIDER

1 tbsp apple juice concentrate
1 stick cinnamon
2 cloves
pinch of dry ginger
slice of orange

Make this in the cup for ease, or double the quantities and make in a saucepan. Place the apple juice concentrate in a cup and pour on boiling water. Add the cloves and stir with the cinnamon stick. Leave to stand for 2-3 minutes. Add the pinch of ginger and the slice of orange just before drinking.

This is a favourite drink for winter weather, and makes a surprisingly good breakfast opener.

NIGHT-TIME SOOTHERS

These make great pre-bed drinks that are substantial enough to be filling, but light enough to leave your sleep untroubled. They are also good for relaxing you and helping you get off to sleep.

Choose goat's, sheep's, soya, rice or oat milk.

RECIPE 1
1 cup milk
1 cup water
1/2 tsp cinnamon
1 cardamom pod – opened to release the seeds
pinch of dry ginger

Heat the milk and water in a saucepan with the cardamom seeds, and bring to the boil. Turn off straight away and stir in the cinnamon and ginger.

RECIPE 2
1 cup milk
1 cup water
1/4 tsp cloves
1/4 tsp caraway

Simmer all the ingredients together in a saucepan for 10-15 minutes to let the flavours infuse wonderfully.

RECIPE 3
1 cup milk
1 cup water
1 peppermint tea bag or bunch of fresh mint leaves
1/4 tsp cinnamon
1/4 tsp peppercorns
1/4 tsp dry ginger

Simmer all the ingredients together in a pan for 20 minutes. Strain and drink straight away.

TIMETABLE NOTES FOR EACH DAY

On rising:
Keep to your early morning routine of breathing exercises, etc.,
Have a Taste Bud Treat
Have breakfast every day

Throughout the day:
Take a drink every two hours
Do not go more than three hours without food
Do not eat anything after 9.00pm
Reward yourself for your achievements and have a non-food treat every day
Go to bed 1/2 hour earlier than usual
Walk for at least five minutes every day

CONGRATULATIONS. You have completed Step 2, so celebrate. Build on your good work and move directly on to Step 3 to settle your system, balance and revitalise it.

STEP THREE -
BALANCING AND
REVITALISING

For this final step of the diet you will regulate your meals and return them to a more conventional timetable. Your food choices will be very specific and geared towards strengthening your system. The work during this phase of the diet is to continue gently cleansing, and to build on the efforts of the previous two weeks. Mung beans become a focus for this work as they provide you with regular protein, and cleanse the gut and the whole pelvic area. Aduki beans are also a very good support for the kidneys – a way of saying thank you to them for all their good work!

This period of regular and repeated meals will speak directly to the part of you that is still missing old habits. The combination of mung beans and lightly cooked vegetables will ensure a full spectrum of nutrients, increasing folates and carotenes, and will enhance their absorption, as well as maintaining a good level of elimination.

Regular grain and vegetable meals also add all the vitamins and minerals you can get from your diet and provide good bulk to reinforce the cleansing, and a sustainable energy to meet all your needs. They will boost your levels of soothing B-vitamins and other essential nutrients.

For the next two weeks you will be eating breakfast, lunch and dinner, and one snack each day if you want or need it. You can choose any of your favourite snacks from Step 2, but the meals need to be made from the selection of food choices on the following pages. Your body will relish a return to the more relaxed programme of slightly larger meals taken less often. Although the range of foods is smaller, do not worry about becoming bored. Step 3 is a gift for the part of you that is missing old habits, and the important part of you that craves security and repetition will feel settled and calmed by it. Any residual cravings or awkwardness you may be feeling will soon be calmed. It will also be a welcome rest from the high stimulation of tastes, flavours, and very regular eating. The selection of delicious relishes, chutneys and condiments will add a real sparkle to your meals.

Each day for the next two weeks your main meal will be based around mung beans, aduki beans or red lentils. Eating these with a grain such as rice or barley, and adding an exciting burst of flavour with a side dish of vegetable or herb chutneys, will meet all your taste and energy needs in a deliciously exciting way. Your other meals can be vegetable based, or you may choose to have a second mung meal to further the good work of these wonderful beans. The more you eat them, the more you will come to love them for the soothing and regulating effect they have on your body. It will not do you any harm whatsoever to eat only mung dinners for the whole of the next two weeks – just see what suits you best.

Breakfast will continue to be an important meal for you, and you can broaden your choices for that meal by including some savoury dishes. Now that you have got a taste for having breakfast, you might be pleased to widen your experience with the choice of buckwheat pancakes. Alternatively, go further and try any of the snack, vegetable or bean recipes, or heat through left-overs from supper the night before.

Keep up the good habit of having something to drink every two hours too. This will keep flushing out your system and supporting the work of your kidneys.

Continue to make meals that are freshly cooked to maximise their goodness. Many of the recipes for chutneys and relishes will keep for up to a week in the fridge, so consider making one each day for a few days and then have a break from preparation while you enjoy the fruits of your earlier labours.

These last two weeks are the seal on top of the very great efforts you will have made in cleansing your system, giving it lashings of instant energy, and addressing a range of nutritional needs. Step 3 will soothe and balance you, and restore calm to your system.

DAYS 14 – 28

You will be working on restoring a sense of calm and balance to your system, while continuing to provide maximum energy and nutrients. Whilst your main meal each day will be based around mung beans, once a week you can substitute red or green lentils, and aduki beans.

• Make sure that you have breakfast every day within one hour of getting up.
• Continue having something to drink every two hours.
• Do not have more than three meals and one snacks each day.
• Make sure that your main meal each day is based around mung beans, (or aduki beans or red or green lentils once a week.).
• Eat a vegetable or herb chutney with each mung meal. Take only a spoonful or so, not enough to overpower the dish, but sufficient to wake up your taste buds and add a sparkle to the meal.
• Eat sprouts at least once a day.
• Eat a sea vegetable every day.

FOODS TO CHOOSE FROM

Vegetables: All your choices from Step 2 including: artichokes, water chestnuts, bamboo shoots, okra and chestnuts (see page 108-9 for previous list)

Fruits: All your choices from Step 2 including: pears, peaches and quince (see page 109 for previous list)]

Sprouts: aduki, alfalfa, chickpeas, buckwheat, fenugreek, mung beans, peas, radish, rye, sunflower seeds

Flowers: nasturtiums, marigolds, cowslips

Grains: barley, couscous, bulghur wheat, buckwheat, millet, oats, rice – wholegrain, short grain brown rice, basmati, wild – rice noodles, rye. Eat wheat in moderation – not more than once every other day, and avoid yeast. This means no regular bread, but pitta, naan, soda, etc. Include oat cakes, rice cakes, crispbreads, crackers, bagels and popadoms, but read the labels to be sure – even some rye breads contain wheat

Beans: aduki beans, black eye beans, chickpeas, mung beans, red and green lentils, green split peas

Nuts and Seeds: caraway, poppy, pumpkin, sesame, sunflower, almond, brazil nuts, walnuts, pecans, pine nuts, unsalted pistachios

Herbs and Spices: basil, bay, dill, oregano, parsley, mint, rosemary, sage, thyme, cinnamon, coriander, cumin, mustard seeds, saffron, turmeric, pepper

Dairy: goat's and sheep's milk, live yoghurt and cheese in small amounts (not more than once every other day), rice, oat, soya and other grain milks daily. If you eat eggs, you can have two a week.

DRINKS

Water (hot and cold) – still, not fizzy
Dilute fresh fruit and vegetable juices
Any drinks from Step 1
Hot Apple Cider (see page 130)
Night-Time Soothers (see page 130)

RECIPES

BREAKFASTS

BARLEY PANCAKES

1/2 cup barley or buckwheat flour
1/2 cup milk (soy, goat or sheep)
1/4 tsp sea salt
4 eggs
1 drizzle of olive oil for cooking

Mix all the ingredients together, beating well with an egg whisk or in the blender to introduce lots of air. Heat the oil in a pan and pour in 1/4 cupfuls of the batter. Turn down the heat and cook gently until the underneath of the pancake is brown, then turn over and cook the other side.

Serve with stewed fruit or a compote, or with a drizzle of honey.

AVOCADO PASTE

1 ripe avocado
1/2 lemon
1/4 tsp salt
1/4 tsp black pepper
1/4 courgette
small bunch coriander
crispbread or toasted bagels to serve

Open the avocado and discard the stone. Mash with a fork into a large bowl, and add the lemon, salt and black pepper. Chop the courgette very finely and add to the dish with the chopped coriander. Mix together and serve straight away.

MUNG RECIPES

SPICY MUNG

1 cup mung beans
4 cups water

Rinse the mung beans then bring to the boil with the water and cook for around 30-40 minutes or until split and tender.

1 tbsp olive oil or ghee
1 tsp black mustard seeds
1 tsp whole cumin seeds
1 inch fresh ginger root, peeled and grated
1/2 tsp turmeric
1/2 tsp Asafoetida
1 clove garlic
1 onion
1/2 tsp salt

Heat the oil or ghee in a saucepan and add the mustard and cumin seeds. When the mustard seeds start to pop, add the Asafoetida and the onions. Cook gently until soft, then add the ginger, turmeric and garlic. Cook for about one minute until well mixed, then add the beans. Cover and cook over a low heat for 10 minutes. Serve with rice, barley, or other grains.

HEARTY MUNG BEAN SOUP

1/2 tsp cumin seeds
1 tsp olive or sunflower oil or ghee
3 oz dried mung beans
2 pints water
1 small carrot
1 stick celery
1/2 courgette or thick slice of marrow
1 further pint of water
1/2 tsp dried cumin powder
1/4 tsp salt

Put the oil or ghee into a saucepan and warm. Add the cumin seeds and cook gently for about a minute until they brown. Add the mung beans, which you have rinsed, and the water. Bring to the boil, then cover and reduce heat to a simmer. Cook for 30 minutes, and then chop the carrot, celery and courgette or marrow, and add these to the pan with another pint of water. Bring back up to the boil, then simmer for a further 10 minutes, or until the vegetables are soft and the beans are split and tender. Stir in the cumin powder and salt, and serve straight away.

This is a simple and delicious meal that can be made more substantial by adding only a 1/4 pint of water with the vegetables, and serving over cooked basmati rice, or a mixture of basmati and wholegrain brown rice.

QUICK AND EASY MUNG SOUP

1 cup mung beans
4 cups water
1 courgette
1 leek
1 turnip
pinch salt
1 tsp ground cumin
1/2 tsp black pepper
small bunch coriander
1 tsp olive oil or ghee

Rinse the mung beans and add them to a saucepan with the water. Bring to the boil and skim away any scum from the surface. Turn down the heat and cover, and cook over a low to medium heat for about 30 minutes or until starting to split and become tender. Chop the courgette, leek and turnip into small pieces and add to the pot. Turn up the heat and cook for a further five minutes or until the vegetables are tender. Remove from the heat, add the ground cumin, salt and black pepper, and leave for a further three minutes to allow the flavours to infuse. Chop the coriander finely, and add to the soup before serving. Drizzle the oil or add the ghee to each dish.

Serve with brown rice for a substantial and hearty meal, or with barley, or basmati rice. Add cubed tofu with the vegetables for extra protein.

ALL-IN-ONE MUNG MEAL

1/2 cup basmati rice or pearl barley
1/4 cup split or whole mung beans
1 tbsp olive oil or ghee
1/2 tsp cumin seeds
1/2 tsp sea salt
1/2 tsp ground cumin
4 cups water

Put the oil or ghee in a saucepan and warm the cumin seeds until lightly browned (about 1-2 minutes). Wash the mung and the rice, and add to the saucepan, cooking for one minute to fully coat in the aromatic oil. Add water and bring to the boil, then cover and simmer over a medium heat for 30 minutes, or until the beans are soft and the dish is thick and broth-like. Add the salt and ground cumin.

Garnish this with some freshly chopped coriander leaves. You can add some diced courgette or other vegetables half way through cooking time, or serve with a vegetable side dish, like a warmed salad.

MUNG DHAL

1 cup split mung beans
4 cups water
1 large slice pumpkin or 1/2 large butternut squash
2 carrots
1 inch piece of fresh ginger root, peeled and grated
2 garlic cloves, peeled and crushed
pinch of salt
1/4 tsp ground black pepper
1 tsp olive oil or ghee

1/2 tsp ground cumin
1/4 tsp ground coriander
1/8 tsp ground ginger

Rinse the split mung well, and add to a saucepan with the water. Cover and cook for about 20 minutes. Peel and slice the pumpkin or squash, and the carrots, and add to the pot, turning up the heat and leaving to cook uncovered over a moderate heat. The liquid should soon be absorbed and the dish will become thick and gloopy as the vegetables cook down. (You can liquidate this for a smoother blend.) Add the ginger and garlic, salt and pepper, cumin and coriander, stirring well. Cook gently for a further five minutes then add the ground ginger and the olive oil or ghee just before serving.

This is a wonderful, high protein dish, that will taste even better if you keep it and serve it again at the next meal. Delicious with plain rice, or any other grain. Serve with a wilted or warmed salad of steamed vegetables.

SPROUTED MUNG STIR-FRY

2 cups sprouted mung beans
1 tbsp olive oil or ghee
1/2 tsp turmeric
1/4 tsp salt
2 tbsp water
1/4 tsp curry powder
1 tsp sugar
1/2 cup mange tout or sugar snap peas

Rinse the sprouts well. Heat the oil in a pan or a wok and add the sprouts, tossing lightly. Add the turmeric, salt and water. Mix well, then cover and cook for 10 minutes over a medium heat. Remove the lid, add the curry powder and sugar, and the mange touts. Cook for a further five minutes.

SPROUTED MUNG WITH GINGER

2 cups sprouted mung beans
1 tbsp olive oil
1 inch piece of fresh ginger root
1 bunch spring onions
small cubes of tofu (about 1/2 cup, depending on taste)
1 tbsp soy sauce (optional)
1/4 cup almonds
1 tsp honey

Rinse the mung sprouts well. Heat the oil in a pan or in a wok, and shred the ginger into fine pieces. Chop the spring onions finely. Add the mung sprouts to the oil, stirring to mix well, then add the ginger. Keep the heat high, and stir often to prevent burning or sticking. Cook for about one minute, then add the spring onions, tofu, soy sauce, if using, and the almonds. Cook for a further minute or so, then remove from the heat and stir in the honey.

VEGETABLE AND HERB ACCOMPANIMENTS

FRESH CORIANDER CHUTNEY

1 large bunch fresh coriander
1/4 cup freshly squeezed lemon juice
1/4 cup water
1/4 cup grated coconut
1/2 tablespoon ginger root, grated
1 tsp honey
1/2 tsp salt
1/4 tsp ground black pepper

Put the coriander in the liquidator with the water and lemon juice and blitz until it is chopped. Add the rest of the ingredients and process until it is a thick paste.

This intensely flavoured accompaniment will brighten up the quietest meals. Add just a tablespoon to each meal, and serve with grains, mung meals, or on pitta bread. This will keep for up to a week.

FRESH MINT CHUTNEY

1 bunch of fresh mint leaves or 3 tablespoons dried
4 dates
1/4 tsp black pepper
1/2 tsp salt
1/4 cup raisins
1 tsp dried cumin
2 tbsp lemon juice

GARLIC AND ONION RELISH

4 large onions
1 head garlic (about 10 cloves)
2 tbsp olive oil
1 tsp black mustard seeds
1/2 tsp allspice
1 inch piece root ginger, peeled and grated
2 tsp lemon or lime juice

Warm the oil and add the mustard seeds. When the pop stir in the garlic and ginger, and then the roughly chopped onions and the allspice. Stir and cook until the onions are lightly browned, then cover the pan and reduce the heat. Cook very slowly for about one hour, stirring occasionally, till the onions thicken and sweeten. Remove from the heat and stir in the juice. You can liquidate this for a smoother effect.

This will keep in the fridge for about four weeks if stored in a sealed jar.

PEACH RELISH

2 tbsp olive oil
2 cloves of garlic, crushed
1 tbsp black mustard seeds
2 onions
2 apples
1 carrot
2 lb peaches
3 tbsp lemon juice and lime juice
1 tbsp apple cider vinegar (Note – this is not on your list of food choices, but the small amount makes a difference to this recipe, and should not adversely influence your success.)
1 tbsp apple juice concentrate or honey
1 tbsp sugar

Heat the oil and add the mustard seeds and crushed garlic. Chop the onions and add to the pan cooking for about a minute to ensure they are well mixed and coated in the aromatic oil. Peel and chop the apples and add to the pot, then shred the carrot and add that too. Chop the peaches and add those with the lemon juice, lime juice, vinegar and sweeteners, bringing the pot up to the boil. Stir constantly for a few minutes until well mixed and the sugar has dissolved, then reduce the heat to low and simmer without a lid for about 45 minutes, until the relish is thick. Stir occasionally to make sure it does not stick.

This will keep in he fridge in a sealed jar for up to three months.

OTHER PULSES

TASTY BLACK EYE BEANS

This wonderfully tasty snack can be eaten on its own with some pitta bread, as a side salad with rice or other grains, or liquidated with 1 tbsp extra oil and lemon juice, and eaten as a dip.

4 oz black eyed beans, soaked overnight, or in boiling water for

two hours
1 onion
1 carrot
1 bay leaf
3 cloves
1 clove garlic
1 tbsp olive oil
1 tbsp lemon juice
Fresh or dried oregano

Place the beans in a saucepan and cover with water. Add the onion and carrot cut in half, the bay leaf and cloves. Bring to the boil, then lower the heat and cover and simmer until soft – around 30 minutes, depending on how well soaked they are. Once ready, drain, and add the finely chopped garlic clove and oregano, then cover with olive oil and lemon juice. Serve straight away.

LENTIL RISSOLES

1 tbsp olive oil or ghee
1 onion
2 sticks celery
2 carrots
1 cup lentils
3 cups water
1 tsp coriander
1/4 tsp black pepper
1/4 tsp sea salt
2 tbsp chopped parsley
2 tbsp chopped coriander
1/4 cup fine oatmeal
1 egg (optional)
2 tbsp oil or ghee for finishing.

Heat the oil and add the chopped onion, celery and carrot. Cook gently until soft, then add the well-rinsed lentils, water, dried coriander pepper and salt. Bring to the boil, then stir and cover and reduce the heat, cooking for nearly an hour. Stir occasionally to make sure it does not stick, and add a little extra water if necessary. The mix needs to be fairly dry. Then add the parsley and coriander leaf, and half the oatmeal, mix in and remove from the heat and let cool.

Shape the mixture into patties with your hands or with two spoons, and coat with the egg and remaining oatmeal, or just roll in the oatmeal. Heat the remaining oil or ghee and when hot, add the patties and cook until browned and crisp on each side.

VEGETABLE DISHES

MINTED COURGETTES

3 courgettes
1 carrot

Cut thin strips from the courgettes using a vegetable peeler, and mix with the finely chopped or shredded carrot. Cover with the mint dressing.

2 tbsp olive oil
3 tsp lemon or lime juice
1 tsp honey or apple juice concentrate
2 tbsp chopped fresh mint leaves
1 tsp chopped fresh oregano
1 tsp freshly ground black pepper

Mix all the ingredients together until slightly thickened. Add a grain or two of salt, to taste, then pour over the vegetables.

This will keep in a fridge for about three days, and makes a wonderful marinade for grilling or baking vegetables. You can also steep the courgettes and carrot in the dressing for up to three hours before eating to intensify the flavour. (Remember to remove from the fridge in good time for you to eat the dish at room temperature.)

WARMED SALAD

> *1 courgette*
> *1 carrot*
> *2 sticks celery*
> *3 asparagus spears*
> *lettuce and endive leaves*
> *1 tbsp olive oil*
> *1 tbsp lemon juice*
> *1/8 tsp each salt and freshly ground black pepper*

Slice the courgette, carrot and celery, and trim the asparagus. Place into a steamer over a pan of boiling water. Cover and cook for 3-5 minutes or until tender, then add the lettuce and endive leaves. Cover and let stand for two minutes while you prepare the dressing. Mix the oil and lemon juice with the salt and pepper, and pour over the wilted and steamed vegetables.

Vary the vegetables according to your tastes and the season. Snow peas or mange touts and spring carrots are a wonderful combination, as are broccoli and water chestnuts, Beetroot and chicory, and fennel, parsnip and squash. Add some radiccio leaves and chopped parsley and cilantro to increase colour and flavour.

SMASHED SWEDE

> *1 swede*
> *4 cups boiling water*
> *1 large potato*
> *1 carrot*
> *1 tbsp olive oil or ghee*
> *1 tsp ground black pepper*
> *1/4 tsp salt*
> *1/8 tsp cinnamon*

Peel and slice the swede and add to the boiling water with the salt. Cook for 10 minutes, then add the chopped potato and the carrot. Cook over a medium heat until all the vegetables are soft –

about a further 10 minutes. Drain the vegetables and mash with a potato masher or blend, adding the oil or ghee, black pepper and cinnamon.

PUDDINGS

FRUIT LEATHER

Make with any stoned fruit – apricots are delicious.

2 lbs apricots
2 tbsp water

Peel the fruit and remove the stones. Put in a large saucepan with the water and bring to the boil, then reduce the heat and cook slowly until most of the liquid is gone. Stir regularly to make sure it does not stick. Remove from the heat and leave to cool. Line a baking tin with silicone or greaseproof paper or foil and pour in the fruit paste. Dry in the oven on its lowest setting with the door slightly ajar until the fruit is dry and no longer feels sticky when you touch it. Cool, then peel away the lining paper, and roll up the 'leather'. Can be stored for up to six months, but never usually lasts more than a few days because it is so delicious.

PEACHES WITH MINT SAUCE

3 peaches
2 mangoes

Slice the peaches, and peel and chop the mangoes. Arrange on a plate and cover with the sauce.

2 passion fruit
1/4 cup pineapple juice
1 tsp sugar or honey
2 tbsp fresh mint

Open the passion fruit and scoop out the seeds. Combine these with the juice and the honey or sugar, and the finely chopped mint leaves.

MINT AND APPLE WHIP

1 lb cooking apples
1 tbsp honey
2 tbsp water
1/2 tsp cinnamon
bunch of fresh mint
5 tbsp natural live yoghurt
1 tsp sugar

Put the water in a pan and add the sliced, peeled apples, honey, cinnamon, and most of the mint. Cover and simmer until soft (about 10-15 minutes). Fish out the mint and mash or blend the apples until smooth. Mix in the yoghurt and extra sugar, and top each helping with a sprig of the remaining uncooked mint.

BAKED APPLES

1 large cooking apple per person
1 tsp clear honey
3 dried figs
3 black raisins
1 tsp ground almonds
1 tsp lemon juice
2 tbsp water
1/2 tsp apple juice concentrate (optional)

Core the apples and enlarge the hollow. Make a shallow cut around the circumference of each apple. Chop the figs and raisins and stuff into the hollow of the apple with the figs and ground almonds. Top with the lemon juice. Put the water and apple juice concentrate (if using) in an oven-proof dish and add the apple. Bake for around 45 minutes in a low to medium oven or until soft.

TIMETABLE NOTES FOR EACH DAY

On rising:
Keep to your early morning routine of breathing exercises, etc.
Have a Taste Bud Treat
Have breakfast every day

Throughout the day:
Take a drink every two hours
Do not go more than three hours without food
Do not eat anything after 9.00pm
Reward yourself for your achievements and have a non-food treat every day
Get up 1/2 hour earlier than usual
Walk for at least five minutes ever day and enjoy another five minutes of exercise
Take your supplements

CONGRATULATIONS. You have reached the end of the *Just Quit!* diet. You have succeeded in following the diet for a month, and will be feeling the benefits on many levels. Keep up the good work – you can return to any aspect of the three steps at any time if you think they will help, but read the chapter on Moving On (see page 165) to see how you can carry on your good work into the rest of your future. Now is a good time to consider your diet for the next few days: you may like to do another Step 1 cleansing, or move on to a wider diet.

Celebrate your success with some real non-food treats, and take some time to plan ahead for the next week so that you can incorporate these into your schedule.

SUPPLEMENTS AND
MEDICINALS

Now is the time to reinforce the good work of your diet, and ensure that any long term nutritional deficiencies are addressed. This will speed healing, restore optimum energy levels and settle your system. Your body will have a lot of immediate healing work to do, and Vitamins C and E are the most helpful for this. The range of B-vitamins are most useful for soothing and restoring your battered nervous system. Manganese is essential along with other trace elements because they are easily destroyed by substance abuse. The vitamins and minerals that your body needs all work in synergy with one another, and it is not wise to supplement with many individual vitamins without addressing the full spectrum of your needs. Most of the nutrients we need are available to us in the food we eat IF, and it is a very big if, they are grown locally and naturally or organically, and we eat them fresh and in the very best condition. Then we need to be able to digest, absorb and benefit from the food, requiring no digestive or absorptive difficulties, and to maintain a healthy gut full of beneficial bacteria, and an absence of any chemical imbalance. So you can see why most of us would benefit from nutritional supplements at some point, just to top up the work of the diet, and that they can be especially useful at times like this, when they can address a range of deficiencies, combat stress and maintain good energy levels.

To supplement your diet and provide additional support during this time of change, it is a good idea to take a multi-vitamin and mineral.

This can be a tablet or capsule, and will need to contain a broad spectrum of the vitamins and minerals that your body needs. There is a wide range available, and you would be advised to look to the more expensive end of the market. With supplements, you tend to get what you pay for. Also, look for the ranges stocked in health food shops or by your natural healthcare practitioner, rather than those on the super-market shelves. Always read the labels. You may not recognise all the ingredients, but the label should show you the names of the vitamins and minerals, how much is contained in each tablet (take care here, because sometimes in small print it will say this is the amount if you take three tablets or more each day) and how much that is as a per-centage of the Recommended Daily Allowance (RDA). What you should not see are familiar ingredients such as sugar (in all its guises including sweeteners), colourings, flavourings and other preserva-tives including hydrogenated oils. Search out a supplement that is yeast-free and that does not use glycerine, lanolin or gelatine. These will usually be marked as 'vegetarian friendly' or similar.

Make sure your chosen supplement contains at least 250 mg Vit-amin C, and the full spectrum of B-vitamins, and that it includes Manganese.

Take your supplement every day, within 10 minutes of eating. Expect to continue taking it for at least a month, and preferably for at least three to give yourself a real fill up. Consider taking another course of between one and three months next winter.

You might want to take the following list with you when you are shopping. Vitamins and minerals are measured using either mil-ligrams (mg) micrograms (mcg) or International Units (IU). You will see that with some the acceptable range is quite wide, but this will act as a good guide in terms of the amounts to look for.

VITAMINS

Vitamin A . . . . 2500 IU
Vitamin B1 . . . . 15-30 mg
Vitamin B2 . . . . 5-15 mg
Vitamin B3 . . . . 10-19 mg
Vitamin B5. . . not yet agreed in UK
Vitamin B6 . . . . 1.8-2.2 mg
Vitamin B12 . . . . 3-50 mcg
Vitamin C . . . . 30-1000 mg
Vitamin D . . . . 100-200 IU
Biotin . . . . 100-300 mcg
Choline . . . . 100-650 mg
Folate . . . . 0.4 mg
Inositol . . . . 100-1000 mg
PABA . . . . 25-100 mg

MINERALS

Calcium. . . . . 500-1200 mg
Copper. . . . . 1-3 mg
Iodine . . . . 150-200 mcg
Magnesium . . . . 150-400 mg
Manganese . . . . 2-5 mg
Phosphorus. . . . . 1.5-2 mg
Potassium . . . . 800-1200 mg
Selenium . . . . 150-800 mcg
Sodium . . . . 250-500 mg
Zinc. . . . . 15 mg

Calcium is an especially important mineral for women, and if your chosen multi-supplement shows less than the desired level, consider supplementing separately.

VITAMIN C

Your need for additional Vitamin C will be enormous at this time. As well as all the fresh fruit and vegetables you will be having if you are following the diet, and the presence of it in your multi-vitamin and mineral supplement, take more. Choose a low dosage of 250 mg, and take this three or four times a day, so that you are increasing your intake by about 1g. If the lowest dose you can find is 500 mg, then take that twice a day, always within 10 minutes of eating. You can take it at the same time as your multi-supplement, but spreading your intake out through the day will benefit your energy levels more.

Many Vitamin C preparations include bioflavonoids. These are elements that are present in nature wherever Vitamin C is found, and they enhance and augment its effectiveness. They will usually be labelled as citrus bioflavonoids, or may be individually named such as Rutin.

Choose a good quality Vitamin C that is free from additives, colourings, sugars, etc. If you prefer, you can use it in powder form, and this can be stirred into diluted fruit juice and taken as a small drink after meals. Resist the fizzy tablets that tend to contain as much colouring and sugar as they do the vitamin. If you take too much Vitamin C the first symptom is increased and loose bowel movements, and if you notice this simply cut down the amount you are supplementing with, and try to increase it slowly once the diarrhoea has passed. It can take a little time for the body to accept high doses of Vitamin C, but persevere because the results are phenomenal. This vitamin is responsible for the health of every cell and blood vessel in your body. It speeds healing and is essential to routine maintenance of every part of you from your teeth and gums to your immune system.

Take your Vitamin C daily for at least the next month, preferably three, and consider taking it for at least the next year. Never just stop taking Vitamin C or it can place tremendous pressures on your body. Reduce your intake slowly, dropping the dose you are taking by half for three to five days, and then by half again for another three to five days.

Also consider buying some Vitamin C and Zinc lozenges. You can suck these to salve and cure a sore or dry throat, and it delivers the vitamin just where it is needed. These are often quite tasty, but will need to be taken as directed on the label – often taking care to have after meals, and not to exceed the stated dose.

DIGESTIVE AIDS

Your digestion will be able to use a little help, and there is a choice of supplements that will support and enhance your ability to break down and assimilate nutrients.

ALOE VERA JUICE is a wonderful salve that gently soothes and treats the whole digestive tract. It can be taken a teaspoonful at a time on its own, or in dilute fruit juice. Take two to three teaspoons before eating, three times a day and experience its cooling, gentle action. This is a perfect supplement for the summer months when its settling action can be most useful, but is the perfect addition at this time of change as well. Choose a juice that is as pure as possible, and expect to see only the addition of a small amount of citric acid as a stabiliser.
If skin eruptions are a problem, bathe the area with neat Aloe Vera juice for a soothing treatment that will accelerate healing.

ACIDOPHILUS is a wonderful introduction of beneficial bacteria to your gut that will help stabilise your energy levels and redress any digestive imbalance. It is especially useful at this time, and can make for a smooth and easy transition into more positive health habits. Choose a dairy-free source, and buy where you see these stored in a fridge. Once home, keep them in your own fridge, and take daily. This supplement is especially useful for women if there is any history of thrush or other yeast infections, and will prove an excellent aid in stabilising appetite surges and settling digestion.

Both Acidophilus and Aloe Vera juice can be taken for the next month. Follow with a two week rest, repeat, and then take for another month later in the year. Return to them if you are aware of any digestive concerns, and always take a month-long course of acidophilus after taking any antibiotics.

HERBS

Herbs can be very effective in supporting your efforts during this key time, and it is a good idea to take these if you feel they will be of benefit. It is important that you do not feel you are popping pills and potions all the time, so if this list seems daunting, take only the multi-vitamin and mineral and the Vitamin C. The rest are optional.

Choose Chamomile, Fennel, Licorice root or Peppermint as Digestif drinks for after meals, and make this one of your new rituals. All of these will have a gentle but encouraging effect on digestion. Vary the herb of your choice, and do not have more than two cups of weak herbal tea a day.

ECHINACEA is profoundly effective at stimulating your immune system and reinforcing your mucus membranes. This can prove a wonderfully effective support at this time, and will backup the work of your multi-vitamin as well as conferring some protection from air-borne pollutants. This is particularly useful during the 'colds and flu' seasons because the work of your own front line defences may need some help. It can take a while for the mouth, throat and bronchi to return to their normal level of responsiveness to attack from invading organisms.

Echinacea can be taken as a herb tea, in tablet form, or most easily and effectively as a tincture. This is an extract of the herb which is preserved, usually in alcohol, and can be bought in small bottles with a dropper that makes taking it very easy indeed. Take 3-5 drops in a small glass of water once a day for three days, then increase to twice a day. Take your doses before eating. If you do not want to take the alcohol, drop into water that has just boiled, and leave for 2-3 minutes before drinking. If you prefer to take a tablet, look for one that does not include colourings, flavourings and any other undesirable or unnecessary ingredients. The tea may be taken as a mild infusion once a day. Take for six days out of seven for 3-6 weeks and then have a three week break. Repeat once or twice during the year, whenever you feel in need of a boost.

PYCNOGENOL is a powerful antioxidant which will maximise the speed of your return to full energy levels and optimum health. It is an extract from the pine tree that has been shown to be extremely efficient in controlling the damage caused by heavy pollution, and will be an effective aid in your progress towards full health. Most readily available in tablet form, take as directed for three weeks, then repeat for another three week course twice more this year. This is most useful for those facing heavy pollution and high levels of external stress. People who live in a city should definitely consider taking it.

AILMENTS

Making such a dramatic change in your lifestyle, however positive, is likely to unsettle your system initially, and it can take a while for you to re-establish yourself and return to full health. It is possible that you will experience some minor common ailments while your body eliminates any toxic residue and works to balance itself. People often experience some a cough, which is the best way the lungs have for clearing themselves, and this is usually a sign that the chest is becoming stronger. This and other symptoms are usually transitory, and can be treated easily and successfully with home remedies. You may experience energy rushes, because your body is freeing up energy for you to use, and this can come as a surprise after stifling your energy for so long. Sometimes ailments just come under the spotlight because you are placing more of an emphasis on your own health, and they will generally disappear once you instigate your good health habits. If you have any major health concerns, or if symptoms persist, consult your healthcare advisor.

Women who are menstruating may notice changes to their cycle, which can be interrupted altogether, or the pattern of bleeding may change. The most common difference is a relief from cramps and bowel congestion, and less bloating and lower back discomfort; bleeding may be heavier than usual, but it is likely to be much less painful. Make sure that you keep warm when you have your period, taking care to keep your feet covered (wear socks in the house) and sit with a hot water bottle for comfort. Have plenty of warm drinks, and nurture yourself. If you are experiencing discomfort, take a herbal tisane of half a teaspoon each of dried Lady's Mantle and Yarrow. Steep them in boiling water for about 30 seconds, and then sip slowly. Take once a day until the symptoms ease. A normal, regular and easier cycle is likely to take a couple of months to re-establish itself.

General changes in the blood chemistry are likely to alter the acidity of the vagina and you may notice increased lubrication and easier arousal. There may also be some vaginal discharge, which can also be a symptom of the body cleansing itself. It should cause no concern provided it is not offensive, or overly irritating, and does not last for more than a few days. Treat straight away by applying some soothing live, natural yoghurt, and consider taking an Acidophilus supplement (see page 155). Adding a small handful of additive-free sea salt to your bath water will help cleanse and rebalance the area.

COUGH

Gently support and encourage your cough by taking a cup of weak celery leaf tea each day. Add a little honey to taste. A warm compress (hold a clean tea-towel under the hot tap, then wring out well) applied to the front of your chest just over your breastbone will soothe and relax you. If the cough is dry and tickly, suck a Vitamin C and Zinc lozenge after meals. The effects of a cough can be very tiring, so make sure you allow yourself extra rest, and plan a few early nights until your chest is cleared.

COLDS

Warm ginger tea will keep your system working and help you feel warm. Bring one tablespoon of coriander seeds and a one inch piece of fresh ginger root that you have sliced and boiled in a pint of water. Cover and simmer for about five minutes, then strain into a cup. Add a slice of lemon and a spoonful of honey, and sip. Drink as much as you like, making each batch up freshly each time. Keep yourself warm and comfortable, and drink more than you eat. Recognise that this is a wonderful way for your body to cleanse itself, and stay positive, focusing on how well you will feel after this clear out.

CONSTIPATION

This is rarely a problem if you are following the diet, but may occur while your body is in transition. Fruit is one of the best looseners for the system, and having a fruit-only day will provide you with plenty of Vitamin C and should put you back on track. Generally, make sure that you are not eating foods or having drinks that are too cold – nothing straight from the fridge – and include warming spices like cumin to your meals to encourage digestion. Remember to drink lots of water.

EAR INFECTION

Have a professional massage therapist work on your trapezius – a huge muscle that runs from your shoulder up your neck and down into your back. Releasing this will usually bring relief from ear problems dramatically quickly. Keep your ear warm, and do not expose yourself to draughts or wind. When relaxing, sit with a hot compress or covered hot water bottle held close to it. Make sure you eat extra garlic.

ENERGY CHANGES

If you feel a rush of energy, get up and do something with it. Take a deep breath, and find a physical outlet for the energy. Simply standing up and taking big, exaggerated breaths as you sweep your arms up over your head and then around to the sides using large, expansive movements will help. If you can take a short walk, run up and down stairs, or do a few exercises, this too will be a good use of the energy. Energy rushes should subside over the first few weeks. A hot cup of something that will let you inhale the steam will be quite settling.

Low energy states should respond quite quickly. For an instant energy lift take Combination B Tissue Salt as directed on the pot. You might also consider checking your daily timetable to make sure that things are as routine and regular as you can make them, and that will help equalise your energy during this transition time. It is certainly worth getting to bed earlier and getting up earlier during this month, and charting the improvement. Ideally, you should try and be in bed by 10pm, and up very early.

Treat cravings by taking a few deep breaths, or drinking a large glass of water or dilute fruit juice. Snack on dried apricots and have carob as occasional treats. Both seem to have a positive effect and disperse any cravings.

HEADACHES

These can be caused when there is a slowing down in the rate of bowel movements, through stress and tension, or just when the body is mobilising toxins faster than you can rid yourself of them. They should be short-lived, and respond well to natural remedies. Make sure your bowel is clear – stewed apple, fig compote, and lemon barley mash are all good breakfast choices that will aid elimination. Walking is the best exercise to encourage this – the mechanical effects on the gut are tremendously useful, and will often be all that is needed to get things moving.

A cold compress (hold a clean cotton tea-towel under the cold tap, and wring it out well) applied to the forehead and another to the back of the neck will help relieve any muscular tension, and soothe and calm. Take a handful of fresh lemon balm leaves and crush them on your forehead for an instant and gentle mood changer that will relieve a muggy headache. Feverfew is a wonderful herb that works to relieve migraines, and a few fresh leaves taken once a week in a sandwich will have a very positive effect. The plant is very easy to grow, and pretty to look at too.

INCREASED URINATION

Keep your lower back warm and well supported – sit with a hot water bottle or an extra cushion for comfort. Drink one cup each day of yarrow herbal tisane, made by putting half a teaspoon of dried yarrow in a tea strainer, and pouring boiling water over it. Leave to steep in your cup for half a minute, then sip slowly. Eat more barley and dry grains like oats and rye. This is likely to be a short-lived response as your body eliminates toxins from your system and adjusts to the diet.

PILES

Onions are wonderfully healing for the lower part of the digestive tract, and making sure you have some gently cooked every day will soon show benefits. (See page 122 for Baked Onion Tray.) The increased Vitamin C level of your diet, and the freedom from irritation from smoking, will soon let your system relax. If the pain from piles is bad, consider holding an ice cube to the area for a moment just before and immediately after each bowel movement. This will numb the area slightly, and encourage a healthier blood flow.

POOR CIRCULATION

Again, this is likely to improve quite dramatically, but you can enhance it by adding a little paprika to your diet, and by using massage. Massage your feet and hands every night and morning, using a light oil if you like, or just your hands. Begin by holding each foot between your hands until you feel the foot starts to warm, then very gently and slowly, use long stroking movements that increase in speed and pressure very gradually. Use round strokes over your heel and up around your ankle, and continue the long sweeping strokes out and off the ends of your toes. Then put on some socks. Massage your hands by using small circular movements with your other hand that work around every joint, and then long running strokes over the long bones. Again finish with long strokes that run from the palm out and off the ends of your fingers.

SINUS CONGESTION

Old fashioned steam inhalations are the best treatment to cleanse and relieve sinus pain. Pour boiling water into a large bowl, and cover with a towel. Sit down comfortably, place the bowl in front of you, and then duck your head under the towel. Breathe as well as you can, and stay there soaking up the warm, comforting steam until it cools. You may need to come up for air a few times, but keep the bowl covered to stop the steam from escaping. Add some fresh rosemary leaves to the water or some sprigs of fresh thyme for their antiseptic and other healing qualities.

SKIN RASHES

Combat and soothe minor eruptions by covering with a paste made from finely chopped fresh coriander leaves. This works dramatically quickly and you are likely to need only one application. Keep it in place in tricky areas by wrapping with a bandage or a clean cotton handkerchief. Apply neat Aloe Vera juice as a wash for ongoing irritations. Dry, flaky skin will respond well to oatmeal – wrap a handful in a cotton handkerchief and tie to the bath tap. Fill the bath with the water running through the oatmeal bag and then let it soak in the water while you bathe. Use the bag to cleanse your skin in place of soap.

Give dry skin a treat by squeezing a Vitamin E capsule on it each day and massaging in slowly with warm hands.

SORE THROAT

Make a weak tea from red sage leaves. If using fresh, fill half a cup with the torn leaves and cover with boiling water, then strain after three minutes. If using dried, steep one teaspoon of the leaves for one minute. Sip half a cup, once a day, and gargle with the other half. Soak a clean cotton handkerchief in some of the liquid, and wrap around your neck when you relax in the evening, or leave on overnight, covered with a towel, for a lasting and soothing pack that is wonderfully relaxing.

SORE AND TIRED EYES

Wash your eyes with an infusion of the herb eyebright. Add one tablespoon of the dried herb to a mug of boiling water and leave to stand for five minutes. Strain and use half to bathe the eyes, soaking some in cotton wool and holding in place over the eye area while you relax. Drink the other half, mixed with an equal amount of water. Used chamomile tea bags that have been cooled make a very soothing eye compress, and slices of cucumber will soothe the eye and help reduce localised puffiness.

VARICOSE VEINS

Increase your Vitamin C and choose a supplement that contains Rutin and bioflavonoids to strengthen your blood vessels. Bathe the affected area with a weak solution of dried lemon balm or crush the fresh leaves directly onto the spot. Make sure that you reduce mechanical pressure by loosening any restrictions (do not wear tight clothing) and assist gravity by spending some time every day with the effected area raised above the level of your heart.

MOVING ON

Congratulate yourself for all your hard work and good efforts over the last month or so. Find a way to give yourself a real treat and celebrate your success. Do something special to mark another new beginning in your life as you set about maintaining your resolve and integrating your new health habits into your everyday routine.

Let the momentum you have gathered in the last month spur you onwards. You may have identified some goals that you can continue working towards, or developed a liking for a more active way of living. Keep working with your feelings and let your body's own emerging voice continue to speak to you. Hear it in your likes and dislikes, your interests, and in your heart's desire. Intention is everything, and your current good will towards your body, coupled with the benefits of the last month, will do a lot to redress earlier pain.

Do not underestimate the value or the enormity of the good thing that you have achieved in distancing yourself from your habit. Find some ways to remind yourself of your achievement that will deepen your resolve not to return to the past, and keep you moving forwards with good health habits. Some people choose to save the money they would have spent and keep it for a special occasion or a treat. You could find a way of marking your success that is meaningful to you.

You can build on this success to realise other personal and professional goals – you now know how strong your will power can be, and how effective you are at meeting your objectives. You will also have experienced the amazing healing power of foods and the strong support that natural remedies and methods can provide. Keep these alive in your life as you continue to express your duty of care to yourself in a positive and loving way. Remember that making time for yourself is a powerful tool that will work to resolve stress and bring harmony to all your dealings. Relaxation skills and regular exercise, breathing techniques and a positive attitude will support the good food choices you make, and reinforce your own self nurturing and nourishment. Remember too, the effectiveness of natural remedies for everyday aches and pains, and consider keeping your own natural first aid kit containing essential oils, supplements and herbs.

Treat yourself to new tastes and ways of cooking but carry the principles of the diet with you. You can return to any part of the diet that you found especially supportive at any time – the cleansing days might be the most useful addition to your ongoing dietary plans. Remember all the good food facts and let them inform your choices as you move on with your life. You will have made many changes to your old diet, and some of the most important ones to continue with are outlined below. If you take nothing else with you, remember the following points:

- Give yourself only the best quality foods and drinks.
- Always have breakfast to provide you with energy for the day
- Drink lots of good water and other neutral liquids to flush your system.
- Eat plenty of fresh fruit and vegetables to give you Vitamin C – this immediate and essential support will aid your resolve and make physical sensations more manageable, as well as continuing the healing work you have already begun.
- Take regular meals – do not go for too long without giving yourself a physical supply of energy.
- Choose warming meals to encourage digestion, and tastes to stimulate your appetite.
- Have occasional rest days for your digestion – choose the juice-only day, or another one of the cleansing days from Step I of the diet. Do this whenever you feel your system getting sluggish, or your metabolism needs a bit of a boost.

A number of the recipes and food choices will transfer to your ongoing diet. As you continue to satisfy your taste buds and move towards a wider and more exciting diet, consider some of these positive health choices:

Reduce:	Substitute
Animal proteins	grain and legume combinations, soya beans, tofu, TVP
Wheat	other grains: corn, oats, millet, rye, soy, potato flour, etc.
Cow's dairy	goat's and sheep's milk products, soy, tofu, almond, rice and coconut milks
Coffee and tea	chicory and herbal-based coffee drinks, herbal teas, dilute juices and warmed juice concentrates
Salt	herbs, fresh and dried, gomasio for a treat, pepper, spices
Margarine/spreads	unsalted butter, olive oil, ghee
Salad dressings	cold-pressed olive oil and lemon juice, whipped tofu
Peanut butters	tahini
Stock cubes	herbs, spices, cornmeal
MSG/preservatives	herbs and spices
Carbonated drinks	dilute fruit and vegetable juices, water, home made drinks, cooled herb and fruit teas
Sweets	fruit, spiced seeds and nuts

FINDING A PRACTITIONER

The treatment choices in this book are all part of the author's training in Natural Healthcare. Natural Healthcare practitioners or Naturopaths, Ayurvedic practitioners and Shamans are among the range of alternatives or parallel choices to visiting your GP. They will all be able to guide you through periods of change and work with you to care for your health. (See page 171 for contacts.)

Word of mouth is a good recommendation, but you should consider the following points when choosing a practitioner:

- That you like them and have confidence in their skills.
- What is their professional training and experience?
- Do they have any areas of special interest that are particularly relevant to you?
- Effectiveness of the approach. It is important to reassess your progress from time to time, and whether you are feeling, and can see, positive change.
- Whether they are easy to see – convenience of their surgery times and location can make it easy to fit in appointments around your own work schedule.
- Fee structure. Most alternative practitioners do not work within the National Health Service. However, many will have a sliding scale of fees to accommodate all income brackets.

All of these factors are important whether you are choosing a practitioner to work with as your primary healthcare provider and advisor, or whether you are looking for someone to massage you or work on your feet. Your body is precious, wonderful, and deserving of the very best you can provide it with, so do not accept anything less than excellence and comfort in all your treatment choices.

THE GIVE-AWAY

This is a spiritual act that is rooted in the early Native American medicine traditions. Essentially it is a way of expressing gratitude for all that you currently have, and for where you are right now in your life. It is a celebration of the abundance of gifts that are truly yours and makes a way of honouring your own life.

In a sense, you have already made your old habit part of your give-away, and now is the perfect time to review whether there might be some other aspects related to it that you can also release and let go of. You might choose to continue the cleansing and give away the ashtrays and other accoutrements connected to your smoking. You could consider giving away some of your time to help others, or just use this as an opportunity to clear your home and your life of any other unnecessary and unwanted things. Another possible choice would be to plant a tree as a gift of clean air and an offering to the planet. Or you could join a choir to let your voice be heard in all its unique sound.

This is a way to celebrate your deliverance or freedom from an addiction or negative behaviour pattern. A chance to express your thanks that something is no longer yours – your addiction was something you felt very connected to, and now you are separated from it. It is a good marker for the transition from the old you to the new you.

Choose a suitable time and place, and make as much or as little of a ceremony of this as feels comfortable to you. Whatever you decide upon, whether it is solitary or shared, intricate and elaborate or a very simple act, as long as it has meaning for you, it will be excellent. It marks your becoming a powerful co-creator in your own future.

RESOURCES

FURTHER READING

Detox Diet Book
Belinda Grant
(Optima, 1992)

Natural Remedies for Common Complaints
Belinda Grant Viagas
(Piatkus, 1995)

As I See It
Betty Balcombe
(Piatkus, 1990)

Where Eagles Fly
Kenneth Meadows
(Element, 1995)

Off the Shelf Natural Remedies
Mark Mayell
(Newleaf, 1992)

Ayurveda
Dr Vasant Lad
(Lotus Press, 1982)

Rhythm and Touch
Anthony P. Arnold
(Brotherhood of Life, USA, 1996)

Do-It-Yourself Shiatsu
Waturo Ohasi
(Japan Publications Inc., 1988)

GETTING IN TOUCH

Association of General Practitioners of Natural Medicine
38 Nigel House
Portpool Lane
London EC1N 7UR

Soil Association
Bristol House
40-56 Victoria Street
Bristol BS1 6BY
Tel: 0117 929 0661

The Faculty of Shamanics
PO Box 300
Potters Bar
Hertfordshire EN6 4LE

Register of Qualified Aromatherapists
52 Barrock Lane
Aldwick
Bognor Regis PO21 4DD

Potters (Herbal Suppliers) Ltd.
Leyland Mill Lane
Wigan WN1 2SB
Tel: 01942 405100

FSC Health and Supplements
Europa Park
Stoneclough Road
Radcliffe
Manchester M26 1GG
Tel: 01204 707420

Lamberts Supplements
1 Lamberts Road
Tunbridge Wells
Kent TN2 3EH
Tel: 01892 554312

British Association for Counselling
1 Regents Park
Rugby
Warwickshire CV21 2PJ
Tel: 01788 578328
www.counselling.co.uk
(list of UK practitioners available)

British Massage Therapy Council
58 Meadow Street
Preston
Lancashire PR1 1TS
Tel: 01772 881063

Dilys Guildford
24 Victoria Road
Dartmouth
South Devon TQ6
(telephone counselling and healing)

ASH - Action on Smoking and Health
102 Clifton Street
London EC2A 4HW
Tel: 0171 739 5902
www.ash.org.uk

Quitline - telephone helpline
Tel: 0800 002200
(lines are open 1-9pm, information pack available)

To contact Belinda Grant Viagas for details of her postal advice service, and for information on lectures, workshops and seminars, write to her at:

PO Box 13386
London NW3 2ZE

Index

Index